Pearls and Pitfalls in
THORACIC
IMAGING

Pearls and Pitfalls in
THORACIC IMAGING

Variants and Other Difficult Diagnoses

Edited by

Thomas Hartman MD

Professor of Radiology
Associate Chair for Education
Mayo Clinic Department of Radiology
Rochester, MN, USA

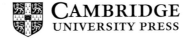

CAMBRIDGE
UNIVERSITY PRESS

CAMBRIDGE UNIVERSITY PRESS
Cambridge, New York, Melbourne, Madrid, Cape Town,
Singapore, São Paulo, Delhi, Tokyo, Mexico City

Cambridge University Press
The Edinburgh Building, Cambridge CB2 8RU, UK

Published in the United States of America by Cambridge University Press, New York

www.cambridge.org
Information on this title: www.cambridge.org/9780521119078

First published 2011

Printed in the United Kingdom at the University Press, Cambridge

A catalog record for this publication is available from the British Library

Library of Congress Cataloging-in-Publication Data

Pearls and pitfalls in thoracic imaging : variants and other difficult diagnoses /
edited by Thomas Hartman.
    p. ;   cm.
  Includes bibliographical references and index.
  ISBN 978-0-521-11907-8 (Hardback)
  1. Chest–Imaging–Case studies.   2. Chest–Diseases–Diagnosis–Case studies.
I. Hartman, Thomas, 1961–   II. Title.
  [DNLM: 1. Thoracic Diseases–diagnosis–Case Reports.   2. Diagnosis, Differential–Case
Reports.   3. Tomography, X-Ray Computed–Case Reports.   WF 975]
  RC941.P43 2011
  617.5′40757–dc22
                                                                                    2011008962

ISBN 978-0-521-11907-8 Hardback

To Mary and Emily, my Pearls.

Contents

Section 7 Pericardium

Section 8 Pleura

Section 9 Diaphragm

Section 10 Lymphatics

Section 11 PET/CT

Section 12 Artifacts

Contributors

John Barlow, MD
Assistant Professor of Radiology, Mayo Clinic Department of Radiology, Rochester, MN, USA

Patrick Eiken, MD
Assistant Professor of Radiology, Mayo Clinic Department of Radiology, Rochester, MN, USA

Thomas Hartman, MD
Professor of Radiology and Associate Chair for Education, Mayo Clinic Department of Radiology, Rochester, MN, USA

John Hildebrandt, MD
Assistant Professor of Radiology, Mayo Clinic Department of Radiology, Rochester, MN, USA

David Levin, MD, PhD
Associate Professor of Radiology, Mayo Clinic Department of Radiology, Rochester, MN, USA

Rebecca Lindell, MD
Assistant Professor of Radiology, Mayo Clinic Department of Radiology, Rochester, MN, USA

Patrick Peller, MD
Assistant Professor of Radiology, Mayo Clinic Department of Radiology, Rochester, MN, USA

Anne-Marie Sykes, MD
Assistant Professor of Radiology, Mayo Clinic Department of Radiology, Rochester, MN, USA

Preface

That's not right, but is it wrong? That question is the rationale behind this book. How often have you been confronted with an image on a thoracic CT exam where you knew it didn't look "normal," but you weren't sure whether it was "abnormal" either? And if it is abnormal, is there a specific diagnosis you should be able to make directly off the images? How many times have you grabbed *Keats* when confronted with a difficult pediatric film and wouldn't it be nice to have a similar reference the next time you had a difficult thoracic CT?

Distinguishing normal variants from rare diseases can be difficult and there isn't really a concise source for that in the thoracic CT literature. This book is designed to fill that niche. Whether it is identifying normal variants that you can ignore or showing pathognomonic images of rare diseases to allow you to make that one in a million diagnosis, this book will give you the guidance you need.

This is not a book of exhaustive differentials for nonspecific findings or a book to teach you to interpret a CT chest or a book of common disease findings. There are plenty of excellent texts on the market for that. This is for the practicing radiologist or radiology resident who is reviewing an exam and has a specific question about the imaging such as:

- Is this a normal variant or an abnormality that I need to be concerned about?
- Is this set of findings specific for an uncommon disease and if so what is the diagnosis?
- Is this set of findings strongly suggestive of a diagnosis and what additional imaging test will allow me to be confident in that diagnosis?
- Could the "abnormality" be due to an artifact mimicking disease and how can I prove that?

Subspecialty radiologists spend a year or more doing a fellowship hoping to see examples of the cases compiled here so that they can add additional value to the image interpretation. Their ability to focus on the minutiae of the imaging in their subspecialty area gives them the confidence to disregard normal variants or recognize the characteristic findings of a rare disease and gives them an advantage over the general radiologist or resident. This book will help to narrow that gap.

This is an image-rich text laid out so that once a potential abnormality is identified, the reader need only identify the region of the abnormality (mediastinum, airway, pulmonary artery, etc.) and then can use the images in that section of the book to help match the finding. Once a matching image is found, the reader can then refer to the heading to see what the diagnosis is: a normal variant, an artifact or a pearl (the one in a million diagnosis).

That's not right, but is it wrong? The answer awaits in the pages of this text.

Tracheal diverticulum/paratracheal air cysts

Thomas Hartman

Imaging description

On CT imaging, collections of extraluminal gas may be present adjacent to the trachea. Most commonly these occur in the right paratracheal region at the level of the thoracic inlet [1–3]. In 8–35% of cases, a connection with the trachea can be observed on CT [1–3]. In cases where the connection is observed, these collections have been termed tracheal diverticula (Figures 1.1 and 1.2). In cases where the connection is not observed, these have been termed paratracheal air cysts (Figure 1.3). However, even when a connection with the trachea cannot be seen on CT, these collections should represent tracheal diverticula.

Importance

Tracheal diverticula typically arise from the right posterolateral wall of the trachea at the level of the thoracic inlet in 98% of the cases [1]. When a focal air collection is observed in this location, tracheal diverticulum should be the diagnosis. This is especially important in cases of trauma as tracheal diverticula occur in approximately 3% of patients and should not be mistaken for traumatic tracheal injury [1].

Typical clinical scenario

Tracheal diverticula are typically an incidental finding in asymptomatic patients. Rarely tracheal diverticula have been associated with cough, infection, or difficult intubation [1].

Differential diagnosis

In the setting of trauma, tracheal diverticulum must be differentiated from a tracheal tear. The classic location of the tracheal diverticulum should be helpful in differentiating it from a traumatic tear. Additionally, the absence of pneumomediastinum favors a tracheal diverticulum. Apical lung herniation is another diagnostic possibility. However, these tend to be much larger air collections and typically cause deviation of the trachea [2, 3]. Additionally, the connection between the apical lung and the paratracheal air collection can be seen on CT confirming the herniation, while with tracheal diverticulum there is not a connection between the lung and the paratracheal air cyst.

Teaching point

A small focal paratracheal air collection in the region of the thoracic inlet along the posterolateral right wall of the trachea is a classic appearance for a tracheal diverticulum. This should not be confused with a tracheal tear, even in the setting of trauma.

REFERENCES

1. Buterbaugh JE, Erly YK. Paratracheal air cysts: a common finding on routine CT examinations of the cervical spine and neck that may mimic pneumomediastinum in patients with traumatic injuries. *AJNR Am J Neuroradiol* 2008; **29**: 1218–1221.

2. Goo JM, Im JG, Ahn JM, et al. Right paratracheal air cysts in the thoracic inlet: clinical and radiologic significance. *AJR Am J Roentgenol* 1999; **173**: 65–70.

3. Tanakaka H, Mor Y, Kurokawa K, et al. Paratracheal air cysts communicating with the trachea: CT findings. *J Thorac Imaging* 1997; **12**: 38–40.

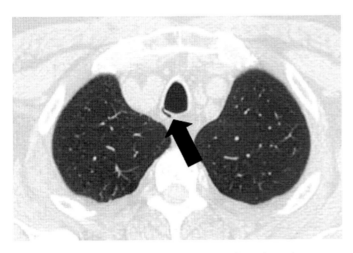

Figure 1.1 Tiny tracheal diverticulum arising from the right posterolateral wall (arrow). The connection to the trachea is visible on this image.

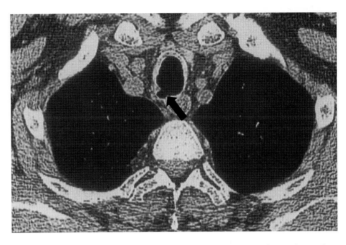

Figure 1.2 Tracheal diverticulum with a wide neck along the right posterolateral wall (arrow).

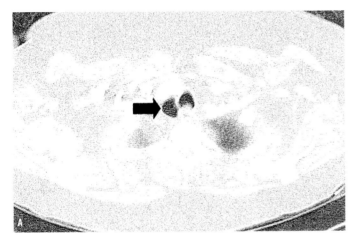

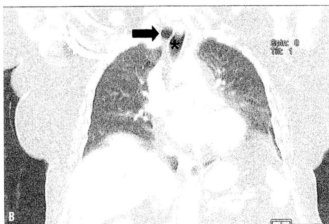

Figure 1.3 A. Larger tracheal diverticulum in the classic location along the right posterolateral wall of the trachea (arrow). The connection to the trachea is not seen on this image. **B.** Coronal CT image showing the tracheal diverticulum (arrow) to the right of the trachea (asterisk).

Tracheal bronchus

Thomas Hartman

Imaging description

Tracheal bronchus is an uncommon anomaly in which an ectopic bronchus arises from the trachea above the carina. It can occur on either side, but is more common on the right. On CT imaging, a bronchus is seen arising from the trachea cephalad to the carina [1–3] (Figures 2.1 and 2.2). This can be easily seen on axial sections, but coronal imaging displays the tracheal bronchus to best advantage (Figure 2.3).

Importance

A tracheal bronchus to the right upper lobe occurs in 0.1–2% of cases and to the left upper lobe in 0.3–1% of cases. Typically a tracheal bronchus is an incidental finding on CT chest in an adult patient and is asymptomatic. However, a tracheal bronchus can be associated with symptoms. When symptomatic, the tracheal bronchus usually presents in childhood [4, 5].

Typical clinical scenario

In asymptomatic cases, the only challenge for the radiologist is recognition of the abnormality. Symptomatic cases typically occur in children and most commonly present with recurrent right upper lobe pneumonia. Other common presentations include stridor and respiratory distress [4, 5]. In cases with recurrent pneumonia, surgical resection is often indicated.

Differential diagnosis

A bronchus arising from the trachea above the level of the carina is by definition a tracheal bronchus if it supplies lung parenchyma. A tracheal diverticulum can arise from the lateral wall of the trachea, but unlike a tracheal bronchus does not supply lung parenchyma and is seen as a blind-ending pouch.

Teaching point

In children with recurrent upper lobe pneumonias, a tracheal bronchus should be excluded as a cause. In asymptomatic cases when a tracheal bronchus is identified, it is usually an incidental finding that requires no further workup or treatment.

REFERENCES
1. Ghaye B, Szapiro D, Fanchamps J-M, Dondelinger RF. Congenital bronchial abnormalities revisited. *Radiographics* 2001; **21**: 105–119.
2. Shipley RT, McLoud TC, Dedrick CG, Shepard JAC. Computed tomography of the tracheal bronchus. *J Comput Assist Tomogr* 1985; **9**: 53–55.
3. Lee KS, Bae WK, Lee BH, et al. Bronchovascular anatomy of the upper lobes: evaluation with thin-section CT. *Radiology* 1991; **181**: 765–772.
4. Middleton RM, Littleton JT, Brickey DA, Picone AL. Obstructed tracheal bronchus as a cause of post-obstructive pneumonia. *J Thorac Imaging* 1995; **10**: 223–224.
5. McLaughlin FJ, Strieder DJ, Harris GBC, Vawter GP, Eraklis AJ. Tracheal bronchus: association with respiratory morbidity in childhood. *J Pediatr* 1985; **106**: 751–755.

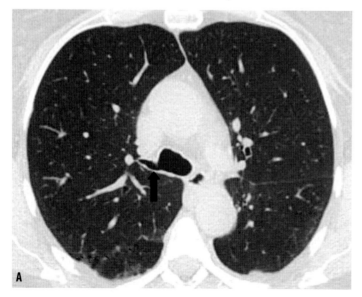 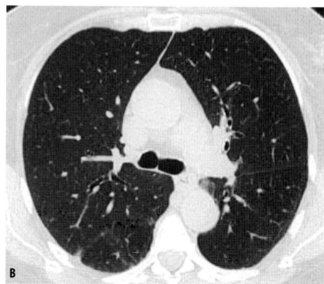

Figure 2.1 A. Tracheal bronchus to the apical segment of the right upper lobe (arrow). **B.** Image 5 mm caudal to Figure 2.1A shows the carina.

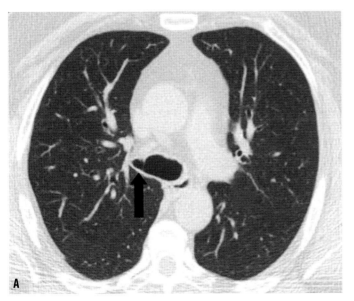 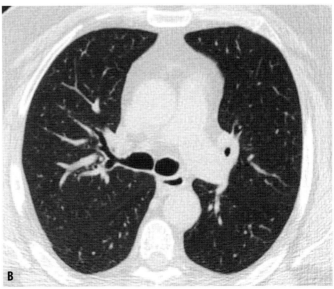

Figure 2.2 A. Tracheal bronchus to the apical segment of the right upper lobe (arrow). **B.** Image 5 mm caudal to Figure 2.2A shows the carina and the anterior and posterior segmental bronchi to the right upper lobe.

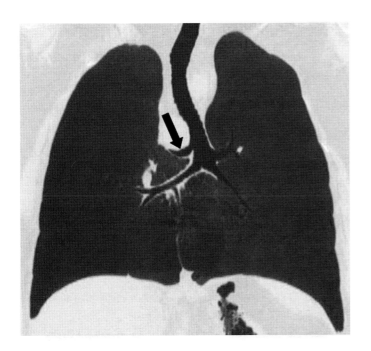

Figure 2.3 Coronal maximum intensity projection image shows an aberrant bronchus to the apical segment of the right upper lobe arising cephalad to the carina (arrow).

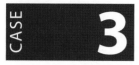

Relapsing polychondritis

Thomas Hartman

Imaging description

Relapsing polychondritis is a multi-system disorder that can involve the cartilage of the external ear, nose, larynx, trachea, and central bronchi. This disorder is characterized by recurrent inflammation and destruction of the cartilage in these areas. Although uncommon at presentation, respiratory tract involvement occurs in up to 50% of patients at some point during the course of the illness [1–4]. Involved airways are typically thickened along the cartilaginous portions of the wall with sparing of the posterior membranous portion of the wall (Figures 3.1 and 3.2). The wall thickening is typically smooth and diffuse [1–4] and often has increased attenuation ranging from subtly increased to obviously calcified [1] (Figure 3.3). In one-third of patients the airways are narrowed. When narrowing is present it may be either diffuse or focal (Figure 3.4). When expiratory imaging is obtained, tracheomalacia and/or bronchomalacia can be seen in over 50% of patients [1, 2] (Figure 3.5).

Importance

Although relapsing polychondritis is a multi-system disorder, airway involvement is a poor prognostic sign and is the leading cause of death in these patients.

Typical clinical scenario

Presenting symptoms with relapsing polychondritis may be seen in extrathoracic areas and include inflammation and destruction of cartilage in the external ear and nose. There may also be a nonerosive seronegative inflammatory arthritis, ocular inflammation, or audiovestibular damage [2, 4]. Respiratory symptoms most commonly include shortness of breath, but as the disease progresses this can progress to respiratory failure.

Differential diagnosis

Smooth diffuse thickening of the cartilaginous portion of the airway walls which demonstrates increased attenuation and spares the posterior membranous portion of the airways is relatively specific for relapsing polychondritis. Tracheopathia osteochondroplastica typically also spares the membranous portion of the airways, however, in this entity, multiple calcified tracheal and bronchial nodules along the cartilaginous portions of the walls are seen and diffuse narrowing is not a typical feature. Tracheobronchial amyloidosis can cause diffuse airway wall thickening, but usually affects the airway wall circumferentially including the membranous portion which is typically spared with relapsing polychondritis.

Teaching point

Diffuse smooth wall thickening of the airways with sparing of the posterior membranous portion should suggest the diagnosis of relapsing polychondritis. The wall thickening is typically high attenuation and may be calcified. If expiratory imaging is obtained tracheomalacia and/or bronchomalacia may be seen in over 50% of the cases.

REFERENCES

1. Behar JV, Choi Y-W, Hartman TE, et al. Relapsing polychondritis affecting the lower respiratory tract. *AJR Am J Roentgenol* 2002; **178**: 173–177.
2. Tillie-LeBlond I, Wallaert B, LeBlond D, et al. Respiratory involvement in relapsing polychondritis: clinical, functional, endoscopic, and radiographic evaluations. *Medicine* 1998; **77**: 168–176.
3. Marom EM, Goodman PC, McAdams HP. Diffuse abnormalities of trachea and main bronchi. *AJR Am J Roentgenol* 2001; **176**: 713–717.
4. Ernst A, Rafeq S, Boiselle P, et al. Relapsing polychondritis and airway involvement. *Chest* 2009; **135**: 1024–1030.

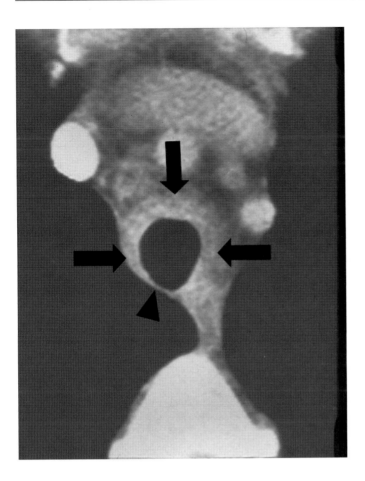

Figure 3.1 Targeted image of the trachea in a case of relapsing polychondritis shows thickening of the anterior and lateral walls of the trachea (arrows) with sparing of the posterior membranous portion (arrowhead).

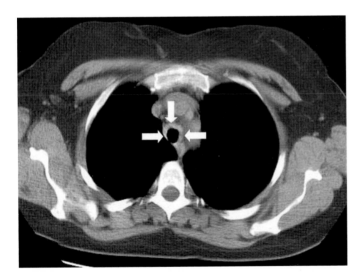

Figure 3.2 Note thickening of the anterior and lateral walls of the trachea (arrows) that spares the posterior membranous portion of the tracheal wall.

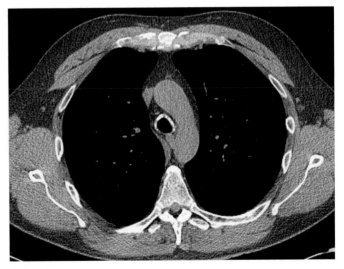

Figure 3.3 Calcified thickening of the anterior and lateral walls of the trachea that spares the posterior membranous portion of the tracheal wall in this case of relapsing polychondritis.

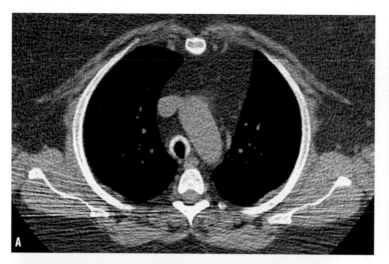

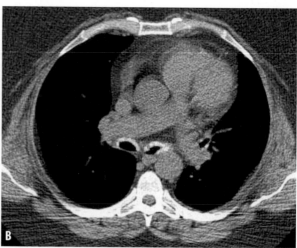

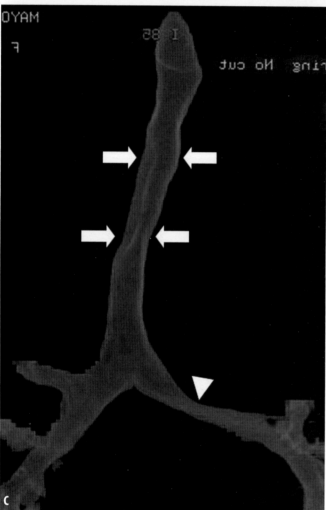

Figure 3.4 A. Calcified thickening of the tracheal wall that spares the posterior membranous portion of the tracheal wall in this case of relapsing polychondritis. Note also the narrowing of the tracheal diameter. **B.** Calcified thickening of the walls of the mainstem bronchi with sparing of the posterior membranous portion of the wall. Note the narrowing of the diameter of the left mainstem bronchus. **C.** Three-dimensional volume rendering of the airways in the patient as in Figures 3.3A and 3.3B shows the long segment narrowing of the trachea (arrows) and the more focal narrowing of the left mainstem bronchus (arrowhead).

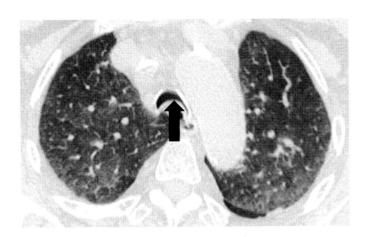

Figure 3.5 Expiratory CT image shows marked anterior bowing of the posterior membranous portion of the tracheal wall compatible with tracheomalacia.

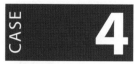

CASE 4

Tracheobronchopathia osteochondroplastica

Thomas Hartman

Imaging description

Tracheobronchopathia osteochondroplastica (TO) is characterized by the presence of osteocartilaginous calcified nodules within the submucosa of the cartilaginous portions of the tracheal and mainstem bronchial walls. On CT, the disease is characterized by the presence of calcified nodular opacities that protrude into the airway lumen resulting in diffuse irregular tracheal narrowing which spares the posterior membranous portion of the airway wall [1–3] (Figures 4.1 and 4.2). Although calcification is typically present, not all lesions will be calcified.

Importance

TO is a rare benign disease that is typically asymptomatic and is often discovered incidentally at imaging. Recognition of the sparing of the posterior membranous portion of the tracheal wall by this process will typically allow exclusion of the other causes of nodular tracheal wall thickening [1–3].

Typical clinical scenario

Although often an incidental finding in asymptomatic patients, when individuals with TO have symptoms they are typically cough, shortness of breath, and hemoptysis [1, 3].

Differential diagnosis

Tracheobronchial amyloidosis and Wegener's granulomatous can cause diffuse nodular thickening of the wall of the central airways and may mimic TO. The nodules in tracheobronchial amyloidosis also may calcify, resulting in a similar appearance to TO. However, neither tracheobronchial amyloidosis nor Wegener's granulomatous characteristically spare the posterior membranous portion of the walls of the tracheal and mainstem bronchi. When present, this sparing should allow

differentiation of TO from these entities [2]. Relapsing polychondritis is an entity that can cause diffuse thickening of the tracheal wall with sparing of the posterior membranous portion of the wall and may have calcification associated with the wall thickening. However, relapsing polychondritis presents with smooth wall thickening, while TO is characterized by nodular thickening, which should allow differentiation of these two entities [2]. Other causes of airway wall calcification such as physiologic changes in the elderly or warfarin therapy typically do not have associated airway wall thickening and narrowing, which again should allow differentiation from TO [2].

Teaching point

The findings of calcified nodular densities protruding into the tracheal lumen causing diffuse irregular narrowing of the airway with sparing of the posterior membranous portion of the walls of the tracheal and mainstem bronchi should allow a diagnosis of tracheobronchopathia osteochondroplastica to be made.

REFERENCES

1. Restrepo S, Pandit M, Villamil MA, et al. Tracheobronchopathia osteochondroplastica: helical CT findings in four cases. *J Thorac Imaging* 2004; **19**: 112–116.
2. Webb EM, Elicker BM, Webb WR. Using CT to diagnose nonneoplastic tracheal abnormalities: appearance of the tracheal wall. *AJR Am J Roentgenol* 2000; **174**: 1315–1321.
3. Mariotta S, Pallone G, Pedicelli G, Bisetti A. Spiral CT and endoscopic findings in a case of tracheobronchopathia osteochondroplastica. *J Comput Assist Tomogr* 1997; **21**: 418–420.

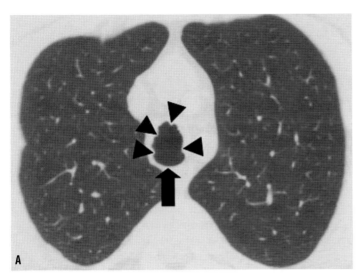
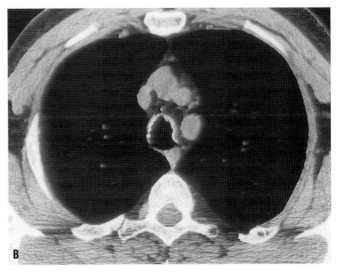

Figure 4.1 A. CT chest with lung windows shows nodularity along the anterior and lateral walls of the trachea (arrowheads) with sparing of the posterior membranous portion (arrow). **B.** CT chest with soft tissue windows near the same level as Figure 4.1A shows calcification in the nodules along the anterior and lateral walls of the trachea.

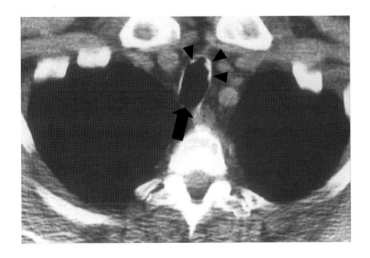

Figure 4.2 CT chest shows calcified nodules along the anterior and left lateral walls of the trachea (arrowheads) with sparing of the posterior membranous portion (arrow).

Tracheobronchomegaly

Thomas Hartman

Imaging description

Tracheobronchomegaly (Mounier-Kuhn syndrome) is characterized by dilatation of the intrathoracic trachea and mainstem bronchi [1–3]. Bronchiectasis involving segmental and subsegmental bronchi may also be present (Figures 5.1 and 5.2). Hyperinflation and/or emphysematous changes in the lung distal to the bronchial dilatation can also be seen (Figure 5.1). Tracheobronchomegaly is characterized by severe atrophy or absence of longitudinal elastic fibers and thinning of the muscularis mucosa within the wall of the trachea and central bronchi. This allows the membranous and cartilaginous portion of the trachea and mainstem bronchi to dilate. Redundant tissue between the cartilaginous rings develops and results in broad protrusions between the cartilaginous rings which can give the wall of the trachea a corrugated appearance (Figure 5.1).

Importance

Tracheobronchomegaly is likely an under-recognized disease as the majority of patients with this abnormality are asymptomatic. This is likely a congenital abnormality that is inherited as an autosomal recessive trait. There is striking male predominance although tracheobronchomegaly has been reported in women.

Typical clinical scenario

Although often an incidental finding in asymptomatic patients, when individuals with tracheobronchomegaly have symptoms they are typically cough with sputum production and repeated episodes of infection [1–3].

Differential diagnosis

Dilatation of the intrathoracic trachea and central bronchi is a relatively specific finding for tracheobronchomegaly. In cases of pulmonary fibrosis from whatever cause, the trachea may be dilated due to traction on the trachea from the surrounding lung, but in these cases the tracheal dilatation is a secondary finding to the pulmonary fibrosis as opposed to being the dominant finding as in tracheobronchomegaly.

Teaching point

Recognition of dilatation of the trachea and central bronchi with or without associated bronchiectasis on CT imaging in the absence of significant pulmonary fibrosis should allow the diagnosis of tracheobronchomegaly to be made.

REFERENCES

1. Woodring JH, Howard RS, Rehm SR. Congenital tracheobronchomegaly (Mounier-Kuhn Syndrome): a report of 10 cases in review of the literature. *J Thorac Imaging* 1991; **6**(2): 1–10.
2. Shin MS, Jackson RM, Ho KJ. Tracheobronchomegaly (Mounier-Kuhn Syndrome): CT diagnosis. *AJR Am J Roentgenol* 1988; **150**: 777–779.
3. Dunne MG, Reiner B. CT features of tracheobronchomegaly. *J Comput Assist Tomogr* 1988; **12**: 388–391.

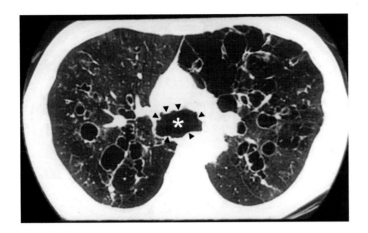

Figure 5.1 Tracheobronchomegaly. Note dilated trachea (asterisk) with corrugated appearance of the tracheal wall due to redundant mucosa (arrowheads). Bilateral bronchiectasis is also present as well as emphysematous changes in the left upper lobe anteriorly.

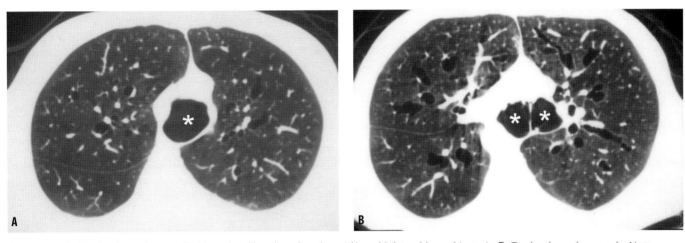

Figure 5.2 A. Tracheobronchomegaly. Note the dilated trachea (asterisk) and bilateral bronchiectasis. **B.** Tracheobronchomegaly. Note dilatation of the mainstem bronchi (asterisk) and bilateral bronchiectasis. Redundant mucosa is seen as nodularity along the anterior wall of the right mainstem bronchus and posterior wall of the left mainstem bronchus.

6 Bronchial atresia

Thomas Hartman

Imaging description

Bronchial atresia is characterized by focal obliteration of a bronchus with normal structures distally [1–3]. Bronchial atresia typically involves the upper lobes with the apicoposterior segment of the left upper lobe being the most common location [2, 3] (Figures 6.1 and 6.2). Bronchial atresia most often affects segmental bronchi, however, lobar or subsegmental bronchi may also be involved (Figure 6.3). Mucus plugging typically forms distal to the stenosis resulting in a branching tubular opacity or bronchocele. There is usually a distinct separation between the mucoid impaction and the hilum. The alveoli distal to the atretic bronchus are ventilated by collateral pathways which results in a region of hyperinflation of the lung distal to the atretic segment which shows air trapping on expiratory imaging.

Importance

Bronchial atresia is typically an incidental finding that is discovered in the second or third decade of life [2]. Recognition of the characteristic findings of bronchial atresia on imaging should allow vascular anomalies or other causes of pulmonary masses to be excluded.

Typical clinical scenario

In the majority of cases, bronchial atresia is discovered incidentally. However, in one-third of cases, individuals may be symptomatic with shortness of breath, cough, asthma, and pneumonia being common presenting symptoms [1–3].

Differential diagnosis

The imaging findings of bronchial atresia are typically characteristic and should allow differentiation from vascular abnormalities and pulmonary masses. When bronchial atresia is located in the lower lobes, careful attention should be paid to the pulmonary vascularity to exclude an arterial supply from the aorta, which would indicate a pulmonary sequestration [1, 2].

Teaching point

When an area of mucoid impaction is identified surrounded by a localized area of hyperinflation with a lack of communication between the mucoid impaction and the hilum, a diagnosis of bronchial atresia can be made. If expiratory imaging is obtained, air trapping can be demonstrated in the lung distal to the atretic segment.

REFERENCES

1. Berrocal T, Madrid C, Novo S, et al. Congential anomalies of the tracheal bronchial tree, lung, and mediastinum: embryology, radiology and pathology. *Radiographics* 2004; **14**: 17–19.
2. Beigelman C, Howarth NR, Chartrand-Lefebvre C, Grenier P. Congenital anomalies of tracheobronchial branching patterns: spiral CT aspects in adults. *Eur Radiol*, 1998; **8**: 79–85.
3. Kinsella D, Sissons G, Williams MP. The radiological imaging of bronchial atresia. *Br J Radiol* 1992; **65**: 681–685.

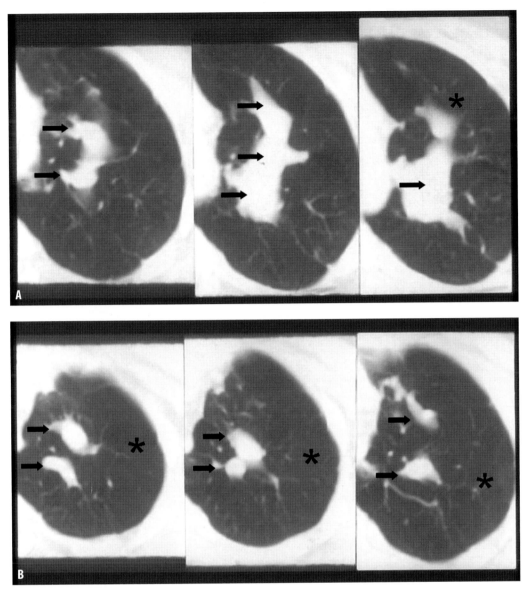

Figure 6.1 A. and **B.** Series of images of the left upper lobe showing the branching tubular opacities of the mucus plugging of the dilated bronchi (arrows) in the left upper lobe distal to the atretic segment. Note the hyperinflation and decreased vascularity in the left upper lobe secondary to air trapping (asterisk).

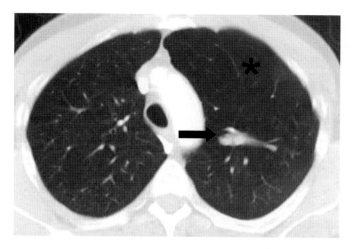

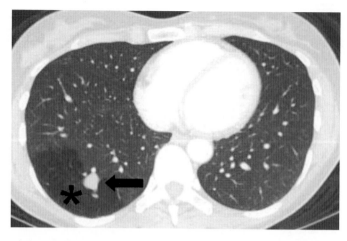

Figure 6.2 Bronchial atresia involving the anterior segmental bronchus to the left upper lobe with mucus plugging (arrow). Note the hyperinflation and decreased vascularity in the anterior segment of the left upper lobe distal to the atretic segment (asterisk).

Figure 6.3 Subsegmental bronchial atresia involving a portion of the lateral basilar segment of the right lower lobe with mucus plugging (arrow) and hyperinflation with decreased vascularity of the lateral basilar segment distal to the atretic segment (asterisk).

Dysmotile cilia syndrome (Kartagener's)

Thomas Hartman

Imaging description

Dysmotile cilia syndrome or primary ciliary dyskinesia (PCD) leads to abnormalities in mucociliary clearance that can result in pulmonary and sinus disease. There can also be an association with abnormalities of thoracoabdominal asymmetry which can lead to heterotaxy or situs inversus. When the triad of situs inversus, bronchiectasis, and sinusitis is present, the syndrome has been named Kartagener's triad (Figure 7.1). CT imaging of PCD shows bronchiectasis with a right middle lobe and lower lobe predominance. There is typically bronchial wall thickening and mucus plugging present as well [1–3]. The bronchiectatic findings are relatively nonspecific, however, when situs inversus is also present the diagnosis of PCD and Kartagener's syndrome can be made (Figure 7.1).

Importance

PCD is a heterogeneous autosomal recessive trait. Therefore, recognition of this abnormality should prompt genetic counseling for the individual and their family. With heterotaxy (situs ambiguus), there are associated cardiac, splenic, hepatic, and vascular abnormalities which should be sought in patients with PCD [1, 3] (Figure 7.2).

Typical clinical scenario

Chronic suppurative airway disease secondary to chronic infection is the predominant presentation in these patients [1–3].

Up to 25% of patients may experience respiratory failure as the disease progresses.

Differential diagnosis

Other potential causes of bronchiectasis would be in the differential and in the absence of situs inversus or heterotaxy, differentiation of PCD would be difficult. However, in the presence of situs inversus, the diagnosis of Kartagener's syndrome should be suggested.

Teaching point

Recognition of bronchiectasis with associated bronchial wall thickening and mucus plugging that is most prominent in the right middle lobe and in the lower lobes should suggest the possibility of PCD. If there is associated situs inversus, the more specific diagnosis of Kartagener's syndrome can be suggested.

REFERENCES

1. Kennedy MP, Noone PG, Leigh MW, et al. High resolution CT of patients with primary ciliary dyskinesia. *AJR Am J Roentgenol* 2007; **188**: 1232–1238.
2. Nadel HR, Stringer DA, Levison H, et al. The immotile cilia syndrome: radiological manifestations. *Radiology* 1985; **154**: 651–655.
3. Reyes de la Rocha S, Pysher TG, Lenoard JC. Dyskinetic cilia syndrome: clinical radiographic and scintigraphic findings. *Pediatr Radiol* 1987; **17**: 97–103.

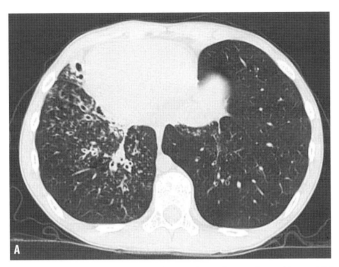 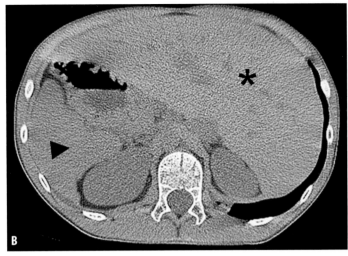

Figure 7.1 A. Kartagener's syndrome. Bronchiectasis and bronchial wall thickening in the right middle and lower lobes. **B.** Image through the upper abdomen in the same patient as Figure 7.1A shows situs inversus with the liver on the left (asterisk) and the spleen on the right (arrowhead).

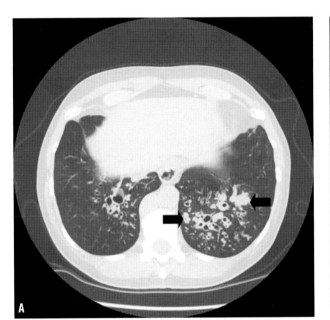 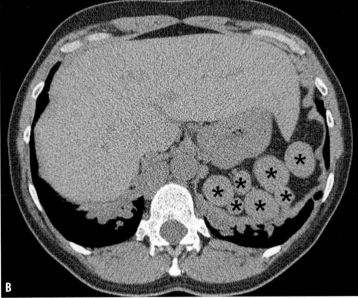

Figure 7.2 A. Dysmotile cilia syndrome with heterotaxy. Bronchiectasis with bronchial wall thickening in the lower lobe bilaterally. Mucus plugging is present in the left lower lobe (arrows). **B.** Image through the upper abdomen in the same patient as in Figure 7.2A shows polysplenia (asterisk).

8 Williams-Campbell syndrome

Thomas Hartman

Imaging

Williams-Campbell syndrome is characterized by cystic bronchiectasis in the fourth to sixth order bronchi [1, 2] (Figure 8.1–8.3). If expiratory images are obtained, collapse of the bronchiectatic segments can be seen [1–3]. Hyperinflation or emphysematous changes may also be seen in the lung distal to the bronchiectatic regions. The cause of the bronchiectasis is due to defective or absent cartilage in the walls of the fourth to sixth order bronchi.

Importance

Williams-Campbell syndrome has been postulated to be a congenital abnormality. At least two separate reports have shown a familial occurrence [3]. Therefore, recognition of this abnormality in a patient should lead to additional investigations of family members.

Typical clinical scenario

The disease most commonly presents in children although several cases of presentation in adults have been reported. Presenting symptoms include cough, wheezing, and recurrent pulmonary infections. Physical exam may reveal a barrel-shaped chest and clubbing. Pulmonary function test shows moderate to severe obstruction [2].

Differential diagnosis

Other causes of bronchiectasis including ciliary dyskinesia, cystic fibrosis, immunoglobulin deficiencies, and allergic bronchopulmonary aspergillosis must be excluded. However, because the bronchiectasis is classically localized to the fourth to sixth order branches, differentiation from other causes of bronchiectasis is usually possible.

Teaching point

Cystic bronchiectasis localized to the fourth to sixth order bronchial branches is characteristic of Williams-Campbell syndrome. Expiratory imaging may show collapse of the bronchiectatic segments.

REFERENCES

1. Watanabe Y, Nishiyama H, Kanayama H, et al. Case report: congenital bronchiectasis due to cartilage deficiency: CT demonstration. *J Comput Assist Tomogr* 1987; **11**: 701–703.
2. Kaneko K, Kudo S, Tashiro M, et al. Case report: computed tomography findings in Williams-Campbell syndrome. *J Thorac Imaging* 1991; **6**: 11–13.
3. Palmer SM, Layish DT, Kussin PS, et al. Lung transplantation for Williams-Campbell syndrome. *Chest* 1998; **113**: 534–537.

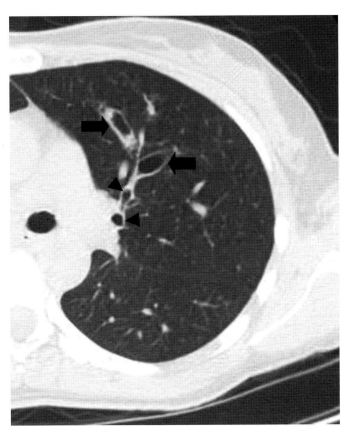

Figure 8.1 Targeted CT of the left lung shows bronchiectasis in the left upper lobe (arrows). Note that the more proximal branches of the left upper lobe bronchi are normal caliber (arrowheads).

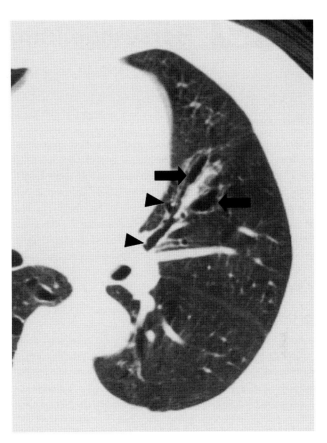

Figure 8.2 Targeted CT of the left lung shows bronchiectasis in the lingula (arrows). Note that the more proximal branches of the lingular bronchi are normal caliber (arrowheads).

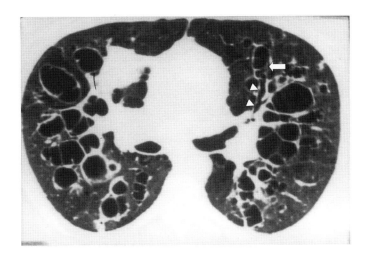

Figure 8.3 CT chest shows bilateral bronchiectasis. Note the lingula bronchus is not dilated for the first two subsegmental branchings (arrowheads), but is dilated more distally (arrow).

Horseshoe lung

Thomas Hartman

Imaging description

Horseshoe lung is a rare congenital malformation characterized by fusion of the posterior basilar segments of the right and left lower lobes through a partial parietal pleural defect. On imaging, this is seen as fusion of the right and left lower lobes posterior to the heart [1–3] (Figure 9.1). The majority of cases of horseshoe lung are associated with right lung hypoplasia and approximately 80% are associated with partial anomalous pulmonary venous return from the right lung to the inferior vena cava or right atrium (Scimitar syndrome) [1–3].

Importance

Horseshoe lung itself is usually asymptomatic, however, there are a number of associated abnormalities that may be symptomatic. As stated previously, the most common associated abnormality is Scimitar syndrome. Absence of a pulmonary artery, pulmonary sling (Figure 9.1), accessory diaphragm, or pulmonary sequestration have also been reported [1–3]. Therefore, when horseshoe lung is identified, careful attention to the remainder of the chest is warranted in an attempt to identify any associated abnormalities.

Typical clinical scenario

When horseshoe lung is an isolated congenital defect it is usually asymptomatic. In symptomatic cases, horseshoe lung is usually diagnosed before one year of age due to pulmonary infection or pulmonary hypertension.

Differential diagnosis

Mediastinal lung herniation from whatever cause can be potentially confused with horseshoe lung. However, with mediastinal lung herniation there are intervening pleural layers in the pulmonary isthmus whereas horseshoe lung involves fusion of the posterior basilar segments of the lower lobes. Therefore, intervening pleural layers should not be seen in cases of horseshoe lung and can be used to differentiate it from mediastinal lung herniation.

Teaching point

Fusion of the posterior basilar segments of the lower lobes posterior to the heart on cross-sectional imaging with the absence of intervening pleural layers is diagnostic of horseshoe lung. When horseshoe lung is discovered, careful attention should be paid to the remainder of the chest to exclude associated congenital abnormalities.

REFERENCES

1. Dupuis C, Rémy J, Rémy-Jardin M, et al. The horseshoe lung: six new cases. *Pediatr Pulmonol* 1994; **17**: 124–130.
2. Goo HW, Kim YH, Co JK, et al. Horseshoe lung: useful angiographic and bronchographic images using multidetector row spiral CT in two infants. *Pediatr Radiol* 2002; **32**: 529–532.
3. McDonald ES, Hartman TE. A rare case of horseshoe lung presenting in adulthood and associated with a pulmonary sling: case report and review of the literature. *J Thorac Imaging* 2010; **25**(3): W97–W99.

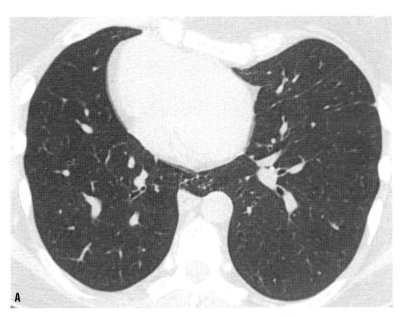

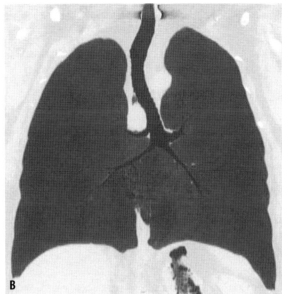

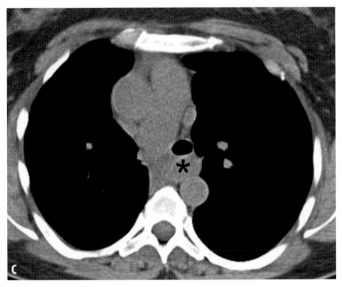

Figure 9.1 A. Horseshoe lung. There is fusion of the right and left lower lobes posterior to the heart without intervening pleura. **B.** Coronal minimum intensity projection image better demonstrates the fusion of the lower lobes medially without intervening pleura. Incidentally noted is tracheal bronchus to the right upper lobe apical segment. **C.** Pulmonary sling. Image from the same patient as in Figures 9.1A and 9.1B shows the left pulmonary artery (asterisk) passing posterior to the trachea.

Sarcoidosis

Thomas Hartman

Imaging description

Pulmonary sarcoidosis is characterized by nodules in a perilymphatic distribution on CT imaging [1–3]. A perilymphatic distribution indicates that the findings are seen along the bronchovascular bundles, the interlobular septa, and along the pleural surfaces [1] (Figures 10.1–10.4). In sarcoidosis, the nodules tend to have a perihilar predominance as well. The nodules may coalesce to form conglomerate masses which result in architectural distortion of the lung. Adenopathy may also be present depending on the stage of the disease (Figure 10.4). Calcification is often present in the nodes and is often amorphous, but can rarely be peripheral (egg-shell). Areas of air trapping can be seen on expiratory imaging in the majority of cases [1]. Additional presentations of pulmonary sarcoidosis include consolidation, cavitation, and fibrosis, but these are less common.

Importance

Sarcoidosis is a systemic granulomatous disease of unknown etiology that commonly affects the lungs. It typically occurs in young adults, but can be seen in older individuals as well [3]. In the appropriate clinical setting, the imaging findings on CT can be diagnostic.

Typical clinical scenario

About half of patients are asymptomatic and discovered incidentally on chest radiographs for other indications. In symptomatic cases, the most common symptoms are cough, dyspnea, and fatigue. Night sweats, weight loss, and erythema nodosum may also be present [3]. The serum angiotensin-converting enzyme level is often elevated.

Differential diagnosis

The imaging findings of sarcoidosis in the chest are usually diagnostic. If the perilymphatic distribution of the nodules is not apparent then pneumoconioses such as silicosis, coal workers, and berylliosis as well as granulomatous infection and metastases are in the differential.

Teaching point

Recognition of the perilymphatic distribution of the nodules should allow the diagnosis of sarcoidosis to be made in the appropriate clinical setting.

REFERENCES
1. Nishino M, Lee KS, Itoh H, Hatabu H. The spectrum of pulmonary sarcoidosis: variations of high-resolution CT findings and clues for specific diagnosis. *Eur J Radiol* 2010; **73**(1): 66–73.
2. Brauner MW, Grenier P, Mompoint D, et al. Pulmonary sarcoidosis: evaluation with high-resolution CT. *Radiology* 1989; **172**(2): 467–471.
3. Criado E, Sánchez M, Ramírez J, et al. Pulmonary sarcoidosis: typical and atypical manifestations at high-resolution CT with pathologic correlation. *Radiographics* 2010; **30**: 1567–1586.

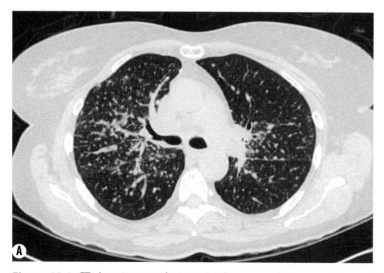
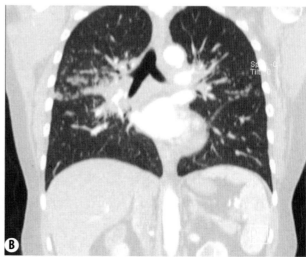

Figure 10.1 CT chest in sarcoidosis. **A.** Axial image and **B.** coronal image show bilateral micronodules in a perilymphatic distribution. Note the nodules also have a predominately perihilar distribution.

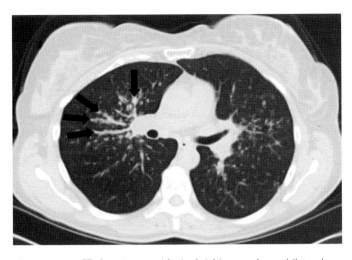

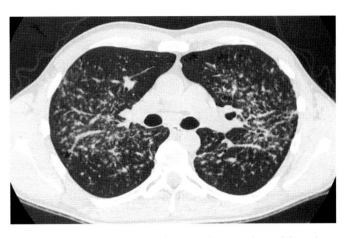

Figure 10.2 CT chest in sarcoidosis. Axial image shows bilateral micronodules in a perilymphatic distribution, most marked in the peribronchovascular regions (arrows). Note the nodules also have a predominately perihilar distribution.

Figure 10.3 CT chest in sarcoidosis. Axial image shows bilateral micronodules in a perilymphatic distribution.

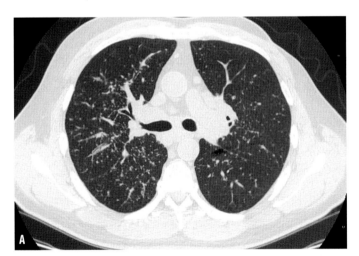

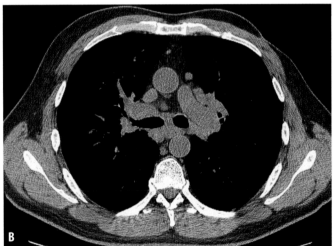

Figure 10.4 CT chest in sarcoidosis. **A.** Lung window shows bilateral micronodules in a perilymphatic distribution. **B.** Soft tissue windows show mediastinal adenopathy.

Lymphangioleiomyomatosis (LAM)

Thomas Hartman

Imaging description

Lymphangioleiomyomatosis (LAM) is characterized on CT imaging by diffuse bilateral thin-walled cysts without a zonal predominance (Figures 11.1 and 11.2) [1–3]. LAM can affect just the lungs, but it can also be a systemic disease. Findings of pulmonary LAM are also seen associated with tuberous sclerosis. When LAM is systemic or associated with tuberous sclerosis additional findings can be present, the most common of which are angiomyolipomas of the kidneys (Figure 11.1) [2]. Adenopathy and dilated cystic masses can be seen in the abdomen and pelvis from obstructed lymphatics (lymphangioleiomyomas) [2]. Lymphatic obstruction can also result in chylous pleural effusions (Figure 11.3). Spontaneous pneumothorax occurs in 20%.

Importance

LAM is a progressive lung disease with a poor prognosis that typically affects women of childbearing age. In the appropriate clinical setting the CT findings are diagnostic.

Typical clinical scenario

LAM almost exclusively affects women of childbearing age. They typically present with progressive shortness of breath although they can present with acute shortness of breath if a spontaneous pneumothorax is the initial event.

Differential diagnosis

The main differential consideration is pulmonary Langerhans cell histiocytosis (PLCH). However, LAM does not have associated nodules, which are typically seen in PLCH.

Additionally, and more importantly from a diagnostic perspective, is that the cysts in PLCH spare the lung bases while in LAM the lungs are diffusely involved with the cystic changes [3]. Other cystic lung diseases such as lymphocytic interstitial pneumonia and Birt-Hogg-Dubé syndrome are significantly less common and have other clinical findings that should allow differentiation. Emphysema can occasionally be mistaken for a cystic lung disease, however, the lack of a wall and the presence of centrilobular core structures (arterioles) within the cystic spaces should allow differentiation [3].

Teaching point

In the appropriate clinical setting, the CT findings of diffuse bilateral thin-walled cysts are diagnostic of LAM. When pulmonary findings of LAM are identified attention should be directed to the kidneys to look for associated angiomyolipomas.

REFERENCES

1. Sherrier RH, Chiles C, Roggli V. Pulmonary lymphangioleiomyomatosis: CT findings. *AJR Am J Roentgenol* 1989; **153**: 937–940.
2. Niku S, Stark P, Levin DL, Friedman PJ. Lymphangioleiomyomatosis: clinical, pathologic, and radiologic manifestations *J Thorac Imaging* 2005; **20**(2): 98–102.
3. Bonelli FS, Hartman TE, Swensen SJ, et al. Accuracy of high-resolution CT in diagnosing lung diseases. *AJR Am J Roentgenol* 1998; **170**: 1507–1512.

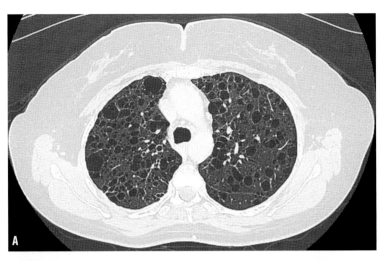

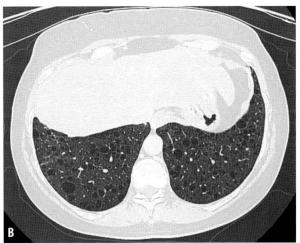

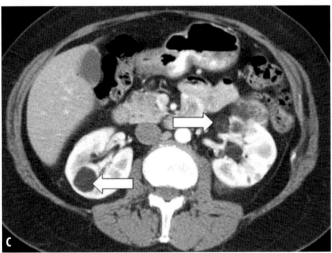

Figure 11.1 A. CT chest of a woman with tuberous sclerosis and LAM. Axial image at the level of the aortic arch shows bilateral thin-walled cysts. **B.** CT chest axial image in the lung bases shows that the thin-walled cysts are diffuse and do not spare the bases. **C.** CT abdomen with contrast shows bilateral fat-containing renal masses compatible with angiomyolipomas (arrows).

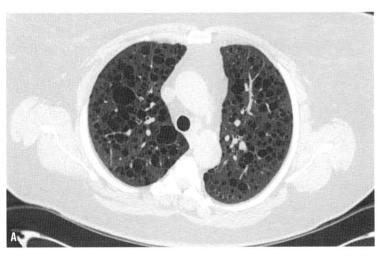

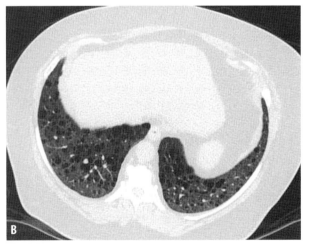

Figure 11.2 CT chest in woman with LAM. **A.** Axial image just below the level of the aortic arch and **B.** axial image in the lung base showing diffuse bilateral thin-walled cysts.

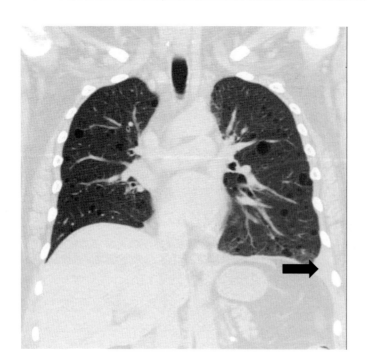

Figure 11.3 CT chest with coronal reconstruction in a woman with LAM shows diffuse bilateral thin-walled cysts. Also note the blunting of the left costophrenic angle by an effusion (arrow) that was later proved to be chylous.

Pulmonary Langerhans cell histiocytosis

David Levin and Thomas Hartman

Imaging description

The classic CT appearance of pulmonary Langerhans cell histiocytosis (PLCH) is a combination of cysts and small nodules [1, 2]. Cysts are the most common finding and nodules are almost always seen in conjunction with cysts. The cysts spare the lung bases (Figures 12.1–12.4) and frequently demonstrate irregular shapes. Cyst walls can range from relatively thick to barely perceptible. The pulmonary nodules are typically 1–5 mm in diameter and also spare the bases. Nodules are typically more numerous in the early stages of the disease (Figure 12.1) while cysts predominate in later stages (Figures 12.2–12.4).

Importance

The diagnosis of PLCH can typically be made solely on the basis of the CT findings. Smoking cessation can result in resolution of the disease.

Typical clinical scenario

PLCH is an uncommon disease affecting primarily young adults, almost all of whom (90–100%) are current smokers [1–3]. Roughly one-quarter of patients will be asymptomatic, with disease identified only by imaging. When present, symptoms are generally mild, even when there is diffuse involvement radiographically. Symptoms include cough, fever, and weight loss [3]. Spontaneous pneumothorax occurs in 10–20% of patients [1, 2].

Differential diagnosis

When nodules are the predominate finding, the primary differential considerations are pneumoconioses, granulomatous diseases (including sarcoidosis), and granulomatous infections. Adenopathy is uncommon with PLCH, in contrast to pneumoconioses and sarcoidosis. Also, the nodules in sarcoidosis have a perilymphatic distribution. Granulomatous infections may cavitate, but do not typically have irregularly shaped cysts. When cysts are the predominate finding, the primary differential consideration is lymphangioleiomyomatosis (LAM). However, LAM is a diffuse cystic lung disease while the cysts in PLCH spare the lung bases. Other cystic lung diseases such as lymphocytic interstitial pneumonia and Birt-Hogg-Dubé have other clinical and/or imaging findings that should allow differentiation.

Teaching point

In a smoker, the combination of upper lung nodules and irregular cysts that spare the lung base is essentially pathognomonic for PLCH.

REFERENCES

1. Abbott GF, Rosado-de-Christenson ML, Franks TJ, Frazier AA, Galvin JR. Pulmonary Langerhans cell histiocytosis. *Radiographics* 2004; **24**: 821–841.
2. Attili AK, Kazerooni EA, Gross BH, et al. Smoking-related interstitial lung disease: radiologic-clinical-pathologic correlation. *Radiographics* 2008; **28**: 1383–1398.
3. Vassallo R, Ryu JH, Colby TV, Hartman T, Limper AH. Pulmonary Langerhans'-cell histiocytosis. *N Engl J Med* 2000; **342**: 1969–1978.

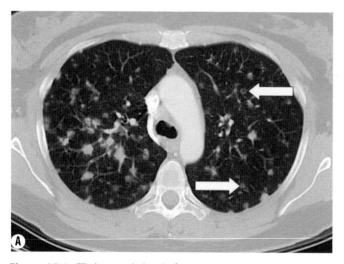 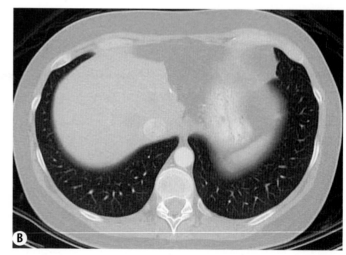

Figure 12.1 CT chest at **A.** level of aortic arch and **B.** lung base in a woman with PLCH shows predominate nodules with a few scattered cysts (arrows) which spare the lung bases (B).

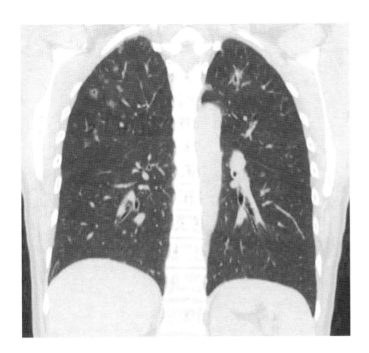

Figure 12.2 CT chest coronal image showing mixed nodules and cysts that spare the lung bases in a woman with PLCH.

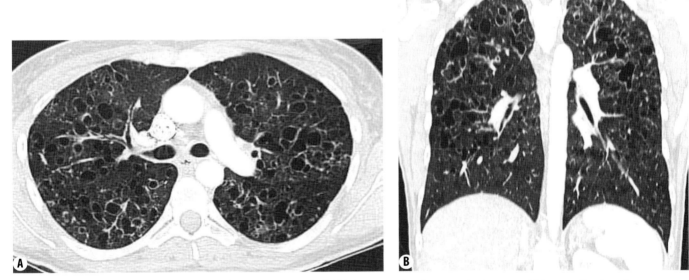

Figure 12.3 CT chest **A.** axial and **B.** coronal in a woman with PLCH shows predominate cystic changes which spare the lung bases on the coronal image.

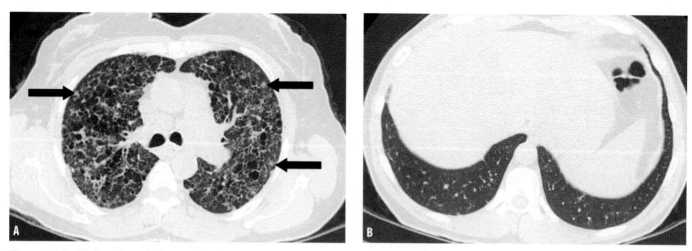

Figure 12.4 CT chest **A.** mid chest and **B.** base in a woman with PLCH shows predominate cystic changes which spare the lung bases **(B)**. A few nodules are present (arrows).

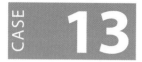

Transbronchial biopsy lung injury

Thomas Hartman

Imaging description

Transbronchial biopsy can be used to make diagnoses on suspected lung disease and can also be used as surveillance in lung transplant patients to detect clinically silent rejection or infection of the transplanted lung. The transbronchial biopsy can result in visible injury to the lung on the chest radiograph or CT [1–3]. The most common finding in transbronchial biopsy lung injury is a pulmonary nodule. The nodule may have a surrounding halo of ground-glass attenuation and may also be cavitated (Figures 13.1 and 13.2). Most commonly only a single nodule is seen, but multiple nodules can be present (Figure 13.3). There can also be associated areas of ground-glass attenuation which may be due to hemorrhage or due to residual fluid from the bronchoalveolar lavage (BAL) that is typically performed in addition to the biopsy. The nodules secondary to transbronchial biopsy can be present for up to 30 days post biopsy [1].

Importance

Nodules are a nonspecific finding on CT chest and can be due to a number of causes. In the setting of lung transplant, the presence of pulmonary nodules would be suggestive of infection. However, it is important to be aware of the clinical history and any recent transbronchial biopsy in order to suggest the possibility of biopsy injury.

Typical clinical scenario

A lung transplant patient presents for routine follow-up or with vague nonspecific symptoms and a transbronchial biopsy and CT chest are ordered for further evaluation. If the transbronchial biopsy is performed prior to the CT chest, the possibility exists that the biopsy lung injury will be detected on the CT chest. Since multiple biopsies are typically performed, multiple nodules may be detected on CT.

Differential diagnosis

In the setting of lung transplant, the most common differential considerations would be infection and rejection. Although, there is no specific finding that will allow differentiation of biopsy injury from these other possibilities, the timing of transbronchial biopsy should allow suggestion of that diagnosis particularly when the biopsy location can be correlated with the location of the nodules seen on CT.

> ## Teaching point
>
> Nodules seen on CT in a lung transplant patient are concerning for infection or rejection. However, correlation with the clinical history of transbronchial biopsy can allow the radiologist to suggest the diagnosis of biopsy lung injury. This can be more confidently suggested when correlation of the nodule location on imaging can be made with the location of the biopsy on the bronchoscopist's note.

REFERENCES

1. Kazerooni EA, Cascade PN, Gross BH. Transplanted lungs: nodules following transbronchial biopsy. *Radiology* 1995; **194**: 209–212.
2. Root JD, Molina PL, Anderson DJ, et al. Pulmonary nodular opacities after transbronchial biopsy in patients with lung transplants. *Radiology* 1992; **184**: 435–436.
3. Daly BD, Martinez FJ, Brunsting LA, et al. High-resolution CT detection of lung lacerations in the transplanted lung after transbronchial biopsy. *J Thorac Imaging* 1994; **6**: 160–165.

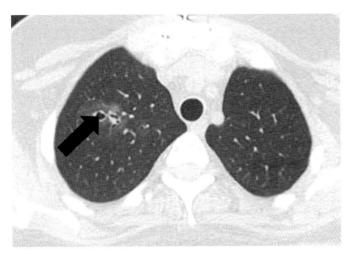

Figure 13.1 CT chest following heart/lung transplant and RUL transbronchial biopsy to exclude rejection. Cavitary lesion (arrow) with surrounding ground-glass attenuation.

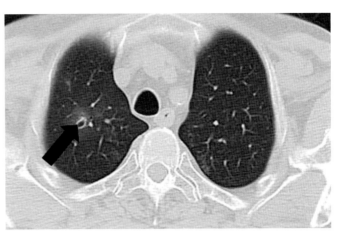

Figure 13.2 CT chest following lung transplant and RUL transbronchial biopsy to exclude rejection. Cavitary lesion (arrow) with surrounding ground-glass attenuation.

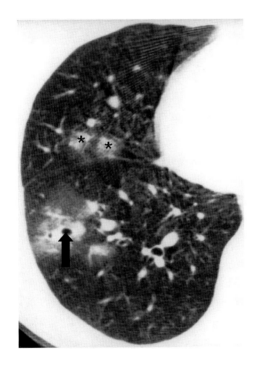

Figure 13.3 CT chest following lung transplant and RML and RLL transbronchial biopsies to exclude rejection. Cavitary lesion (arrow) with surrounding ground-glass attenuation. There is also nodular ground-glass attenuation in the right middle lobe (asterisks) likely secondary to biopsy changes.

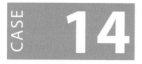

CASE 14

Congenital cystic adenomatoid malformation

David Levin and Thomas Hartman

Imaging description

Congenital cystic adenomatoid malformations (CCAMs) account for 25% of all congenital lung abnormalities. CCAMs are divided into three types: type 1 consists of cysts between 2 cm and 10 cm in diameter; type 2 consists of cysts between 0.5 cm and 2 cm in diameter; and type 3 consists of microscopic cysts [1–3]. Most lesions are identified within the first two years of life. However, in the rare cases where the lesions are not identified until adulthood, they are usually either type 1 or type 2 CCAMs. On imaging, type 1 CCAMs are most commonly a large cyst (up to 12 cm in diameter) or a few cysts, possibly containing air/fluid levels. Type 2 CCAMs are typically multicystic (2–20 mm in diameter) and may also contain air/fluid levels (Figure 14.1). CCAMs typically exhibit mass effect on the adjacent lung and when large enough can displace mediastinal structures. They are most commonly seen in the lower lobes and are surrounded by "normal" lung parenchyma.

Importance

CCAMs are a common congenital lesion of the lung and should be considered in the differential of pulmonary lesions detected in early childhood or prenatally. In the adult, the lesions are a cause of recurrent infection.

Typical clinical scenario

CCAMs typically present during the neonatal period as large, expanding, parenchymal mass lesions associated with respiratory distress. In adulthood, CCAMs may present as cystic lesions in patients with recurrent pneumonias.

Differential diagnosis

In the adult patient, the differential includes cystic bronchiectasis, pneumatocele, intrapulmonary sequestration, and intrapulmonary bronchogenic cyst. Type 1 CCAMs can have some imaging overlap with bronchogenic cysts, however, the imaging findings for type 2 CCAMs should allow the diagnosis.

Teaching point

CCAMs are a common pulmonary lesion in the prenatal and early childhood periods, but can be encountered in the adult. The imaging features will depend on the type of CCAM encountered. The diagnosis of a type 2 CCAM in an adult can usually be made based on the imaging findings.

REFERENCES

1. Rosado de Christenson ML, Stocker JT. Congenital cystic adenomatoid malformation. *Radiographics* 1991; **11**: 865–886.
2. Zylak CJ, Eyler WR, Spizarny DL, Stone CH. Developmental lung anomalies in the adult: radiologic-pathologic correlation. *Radiographics* 2002; **22**: S25–S43.
3. Patz EF Jr, Müller NL, Swensen SJ, Dodd LG. Congenital cystic adenomatoid malformation in adults: CT findings. *J Comput Assist Tomogr* 1995; **19**: 361–364.

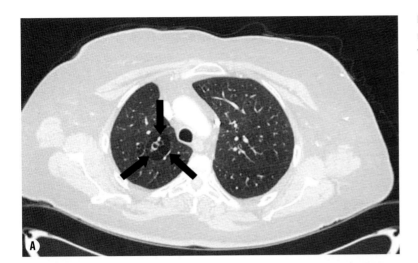

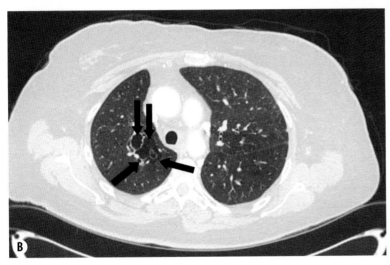

Figure 14.1 **A.** and **B.** Enhanced CT at two levels shows a multicystic lesion (CCAM) in the right upper lobe with variable-sized air cysts within the lesion (arrows).

Lymphocytic interstitial pneumonia

David Levin and Thomas Hartman

Imaging description

The primary imaging findings of lymphocytic interstitial pneumonia (LIP) are bilateral regions of ground-glass opacity [1, 2]. These are most often diffuse, but may be patchy in distribution. Most patients will also have poorly defined centrilobular nodules. Thickening of interlobular septa and bronchovascular bundles is present in 80% of patients. Small subpleural nodules are also seen in nearly 80% of patients. Parenchymal cysts are present in roughly two-thirds of all patients (Figures 15.1 and 15.2). Pleural effusions are rare.

Importance

Lymphocytic interstitial pneumonia in the adult is a benign disorder characterized by infiltration of the pulmonary interstitium by lymphocytes and plasma cells [1, 2]. LIP is characteristically steroid responsive.

Typical clinical scenario

LIP is most often associated with other systemic disease, such as Sjogren's syndrome, HIV infection in children, autoimmune thyroid disorders, and multicentric Castleman's disease. Symptoms are usually slowly progressive and include cough, dyspnea, and fevers.

Differential diagnosis

The findings of LIP are nonspecific and can be seen with a number of other disease processes, including atypical infections and edema. However, the identification of parenchymal cysts and subpleural nodules in addition to the areas of ground-glass attenuation strongly favors the diagnosis of LIP (Figures 15.1 and 15.2).

Teaching point

In the setting of Sjogren's syndrome, the presence of ground-glass opacities and/or poorly defined centrilobular nodules with additional findings of air cysts, plus or minus subpleural nodules and interlobular septal thickening should suggest the diagnosis of LIP.

REFERENCES

1. Honda O, Johkoh T, Ichikado K, et al. Differential diagnosis of lymphocytic interstitial pneumonia and malignant lymphoma on high-resolution CT. *AJR Am J Roentgenol* 1999; **173**(1): 71–74.
2. Johkoh T, Muller NL, Pickford HA, et al. Lymphocytic interstitial pneumonia: thin-section CT findings in 22 patients. *Radiology* 1999; **212**(2): 567–572.

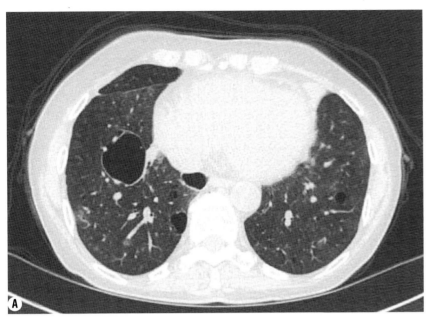
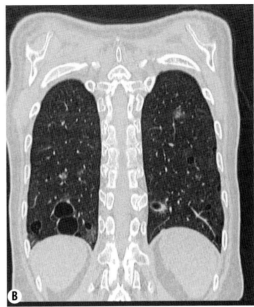

Figure 15.1 CT chest **A.** axial and **B.** coronal images of LIP in a patient with Sjogren's syndrome show bilateral areas of scattered ground-glass attenuation and air cysts of varying sizes with a lower lung predominance.

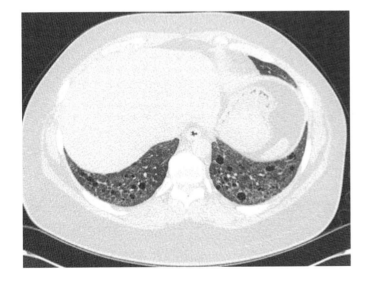

Figure 15.2 CT chest in a patient with Sjogren's syndrome shows more confluent areas of ground-glass attenuation with scattered air cysts in the lower lungs in this patient with LIP.

Intralobar sequestration

David Levin and Thomas Hartman

Imaging description

Pulmonary sequestration is uncommon and can be divided into intralobar and extralobar types, depending on specific morphologic features. In general terms, sequestration refers to lung tissue that is isolated from the tracheobronchial tree [1–3]. Intralobar sequestration accounts for 75% of all pulmonary sequestration and consists of an abnormal segment of lung located within otherwise normal lung. Blood supply is via anomalous systemic vessels arising from the aorta (Figures 16.1–16.3), which typically travel within the inferior pulmonary ligament [1–3]. Most intralobar sequestrations are drained by normal pulmonary veins into the left atrium. Intralobar sequestration typically occurs within the lower lobes, more frequently on the left. Air-bronchograms, bronchiectasis, or cavitation can be seen. Although cases can be congenital, most cases are acquired, likely on the basis of early childhood infection.

Importance

Intralobar sequestrations are a cause of recurrent infections and while uncommon, the imaging features allow for a specific diagnosis. Recognition of the anomalous systemic vessels is also important when resection is planned.

Typical clinical scenario

Intralobar sequestration is typically diagnosed in early adulthood. Most patients are symptomatic, with chronic cough, sputum, recurrent pneumonia, or hemoptysis. Males and females are equally affected.

Differential diagnosis

The typical radiographic appearance is a homogeneous region of consolidation with smooth or lobulated borders. The differential diagnosis would include a focus of recurrent or nonresolving pneumonia, aspiration, organizing pneumonia, or neoplasm.

Teaching point

Intralobar sequestration, while uncommon, should be considered when a region of persistent focal consolidation is identified, especially when it occurs within the lower lobes. The identification of a systemic vascular supply confirms the diagnosis.

REFERENCES

1. Frazier AA, Rosado de Christenson ML, Stocker JT, Templeton PA. Intralobar sequestration: radiologic-pathologic correlation. *Radiographics* 1997; **17**: 725–745.
2. Zylak CJ, Eyler WR, Spizarny DL, Stone CH. Developmental lung anomalies in the adult: radiologic-pathologic correlation. *Radiographics* 2002; **22**: S25–S43.
3. Rappaport DC, Herman S, Weisbrod G. Congenital bronchopulmonary diseases in adults: CT findings. *AJR Am J Roentgenol* 1994; **162**: 1295–1299.

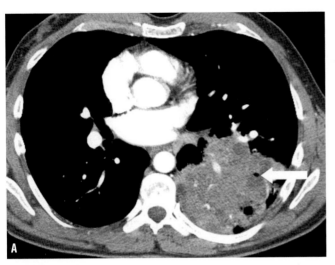 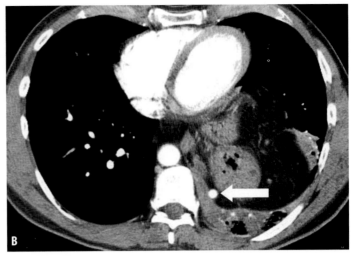

Figure 16.1 Intralobar sequestration. **A.** Contrast-enhanced CT showing an irregular area of consolidation in the left lower lobe with air/fluid level (arrow). **B.** Image lower in the chest shows the large anomalous arterial supply to the sequestration (arrow) that arose from the celiac axis. Elevation of left hemidiaphragm was also present.

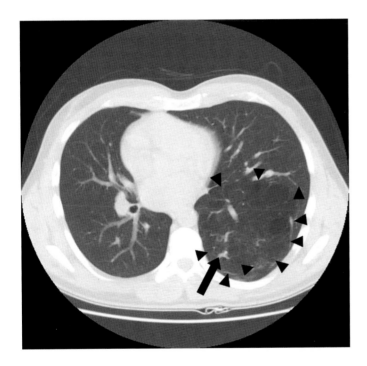

Figure 16.2 Intralobar sequestration from the same patient as Figure 16.1 prior to the infection of the sequestration. Note the multiple irregular airspaces of the lesion (arrowheads) and the irregular vessel with abnormal orientation in the left lower lobe posteromedially which is the anomalous arterial supply (arrow).

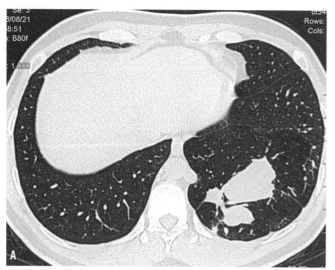

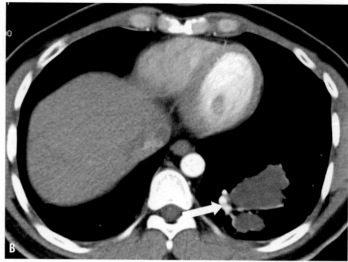

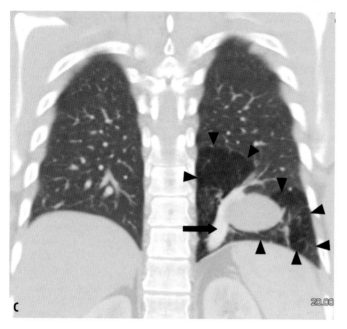

Figure 16.3 CT chest of intralobar sequestration. **A.** Lung windows, **B.** soft tissue windows, and **C.** coronal maximum intensity projection (MIP) reconstructed image with lung windows. Multifocal consolidation in the left lower lobe with a large anomalous vessel along the medial aspect of the consolidation (arrows). This vessel is seen to course inferomedially on the MIP image and eventually this vessel connected with the aorta. The extent of the sequestration is better appreciated on the MIP image as the area of decreased attenuation and vascularity (arrowheads) that extend beyond just the consolidated portion.

Erdheim-Chester disease

David Levin and Anne-Marie Sykes

Imaging description

Erdheim-Chester disease is a very rare interstitial lung disease characterized by infiltration of non-Langerhans cell histiocytes or macrophages forming granulomatous lesions with fibrosis. The bones are the primary site of involvement (osteosclerotic lesions) (Figures 17.1 and 17.2), but pulmonary involvement can occur. The infiltration occurs most prominently along the lymphatics, and therefore affects the interlobular septa, bronchovascular bundles, and visceral pleura. On high-resolution CT chest, the major findings are smooth thickening of the fissures and interlobular septa, ground-glass opacities, and centrilobular nodules, which are slightly more prominent in the mid and upper lungs (Figures 17.1–17.3) [1–3]. Pleural effusions are present in roughly 50% of cases (Figure 17.1). Other common findings include pericardial thickening or effusion and extrathoracic soft tissue masses. The extrathoracic soft tissue is often seen surrounding the kidneys and in the retroperitoneum (Figures 17.2 and 17.3) [2].

Importance

Although pulmonary involvement with Erdheim-Chester disease is uncommon, the resulting lung disease is associated with significant morbidity and mortality. Radiographic evidence of disease often precedes clinical symptoms [2].

Typical clinical scenario

Patients most commonly present with bone pain, particularly involving the lower limbs. Respiratory symptoms include dyspnea and cough. Pulmonary function tests often reveal moderate restrictive defects with a decreased diffusion capacity. There may be mild-to-moderate hypoxemia. Exophthalmos and diabetes insipidus can also be seen.

Differential diagnosis

Initial CT chest examination may raise the question of congestive heart failure (CHF) with interstitial edema, although centrilobular nodules are not typically seen with CHF. Lymphangitic metastases result in interstitial thickening, but the thickening is usually nodular. The septal thickening in pulmonary lymphangiomatosis also affects bronchovascular bundles, but is associated with infiltration of mediastinal fat. Pulmonary veno-occlusive disease results in interstitial thickening and ground-glass opacities, but typically also has enlarged central pulmonary arteries.

> ## Teaching point
>
> Erdheim-Chester disease should be diagnosed in a patient who has the combination of bone pain, osteosclerotic lesions, and CT chest findings of septal thickening, reticular and ground-glass opacities, and centrilobular nodules.

REFERENCES

1. Hansell DM, Armstrong P, Lynch DA, McAdams HP. *Imaging of Diseases of the Chest*, 4th edn. Philadelphia, PA: Elsevier Mosby 2005; 686.
2. Wittenberg KH, Swensen SJ, Myers JL. Pulmonary involvement with Erdheim Chester disease: radiographic and CT findings. *AJR Am J Roentgenol* 2000; **174**: 1327–1331.
3. Dion E, Graef C, Haroche J, et al. Imaging of thoracoabdominal involvement in Erdheim–Chester disease. *AJR Am J Roentgenol* 2004; **183**: 1253–1260.

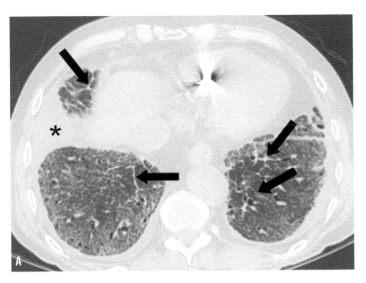

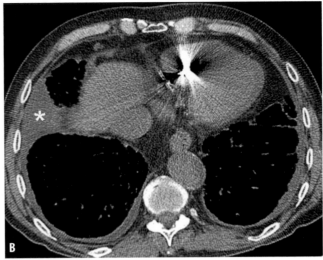

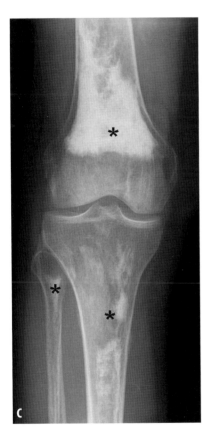

Figure 17.1 A. CT chest without contrast. Lung windows show bilateral areas of ground-glass attenuation with associated interlobular septal thickening (arrows). There is a small right pleural effusion (asterisk). **B.** CT chest without contrast from same level as Figure 17.1A. Soft tissue windows show a right pleural effusion (asterisk). There was infiltrating soft tissue in the renal hilum bilaterally (not shown). **C.** Radiograph of the right knee in the same patient as in Figures 17.1A and 17.1B showing dense sclerosis in the distal femur, proximal tibia, and proximal fibula (asterisks) compatible with Erdheim-Chester disease. Similar findings were present on the left (not shown).

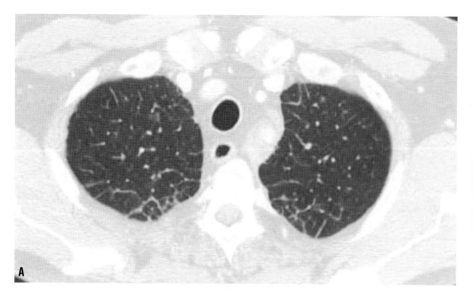

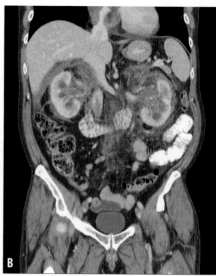

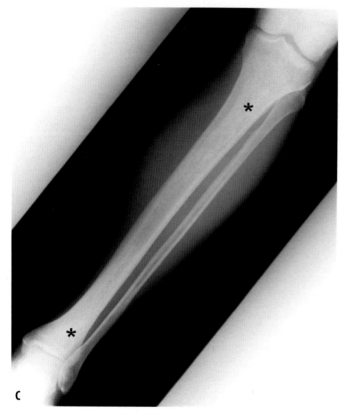

Figure 17.2 A. CT chest with contrast. Lung windows show bilateral nodular areas of ground-glass attenuation with associated interlobular septal thickening. **B.** CT abdomen coronal image with contrast in the same patient as in Figure 17.2A shows infiltrating soft tissue surrounding the kidneys and in the retroperitoneum. This soft tissue is compatible with extrapulmonary Erdheim-Chester disease. **C.** Radiograph of the left tibia and fibula in the same patient as in Figures 17.2A and 17.2B showing sclerosis in the proximal and distal tibia (asterisks) with Erdheim-Chester disease Similar findings were present on the right (not shown).

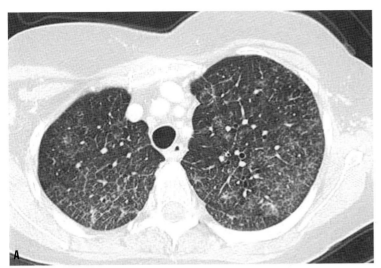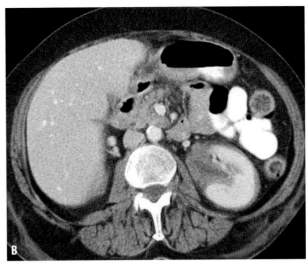

Figure 17.3 A. CT chest with contrast. Lung windows shows bilateral areas of ground-glass attenuation with associated interlobular septal thickening. B. CT abdomen with contrast in the same patient as in Figure 17.3A shows infiltrating soft tissue surrounding the left kidney. Although nonspecific, this soft tissue is compatible with extrapulmonary Erdheim-Chester disease. Similar soft tissue was seen surrounding the right kidney (not shown).

Exogenous lipoid pneumonia

David Levin and Thomas Hartman

Imaging description

The typical imaging findings of exogenous lipoid pneumonia consist of bilateral foci of patchy consolidation and ground-glass opacity. The lung bases are most commonly involved. The regions of consolidation are frequently of decreased attenuation and may have attenuation values consistent with fat [1–3] (Figures 18.1 and 18.2). A "crazy-paving" pattern of ground-glass opacity and septal thickening has also been reported in patients with exogenous lipoid pneumonia [1–3] (Figure 18.3).

Importance

The imaging appearance is often diagnostic and should prompt further clinical evaluation for a source of the exogenous lipoid material.

Typical clinical scenario

Exogenous lipoid pneumonia is an uncommon disease caused by the aspiration or inhalation of oils or other fatty substances. Most cases occur as a result of aspiration of paraffin oil, which can be used as a laxative. Rarely, cases can occur as a result of occupational exposure from industrial lubricants and cutting fluids [1, 2]. Most individuals are asymptomatic, but when present, the most common clinical symptoms are cough and dyspnea [1, 2].

Differential diagnosis

The finding of fat attenuation consolidation is diagnostic of exogenous lipoid pneumonia. The crazy-paving pattern of ground-glass opacity has a broad differential, including pulmonary alveolar proteinosis, infection, hemorrhage, and edema.

Teaching point

The classic appearance of exogenous lipoid pneumonia is bilateral regions of fat attenuation consolidation in the dependent portions of the lung.

REFERENCES

1. Betancourt SL, Martinez-Jimenez S, Rossi SE, et al. Lipoid pneumonia: spectrum of clinical and radiologic manifestations *AJR Am J Roentgenol* 2010; **194**: 103–109.
2. Baron SE, Haramati LB, Rivera VT. Radiological and clinical findings in acute and chronic exogenous lipoid pneumonia. *J Thorac Imaging* 2003; **18**: 217–224.
3. Franquet T, Giménez A, Bordes R, Rodriguez-Arias JM, Castella J. The crazy paving pattern in exogenous lipoid pneumonia: CT-pathologic correlation. *AJR Am J Roentgenol* 1998; **170**: 315–317.

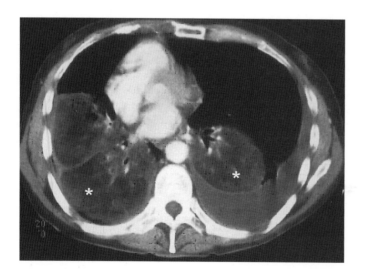

Figure 18.1 Contrast-enhanced CT shows bilateral areas of consolidation (asterisks) with a left pleural effusion. The consolidation is fat attenuation and confirms the diagnosis of lipoid pneumonia.

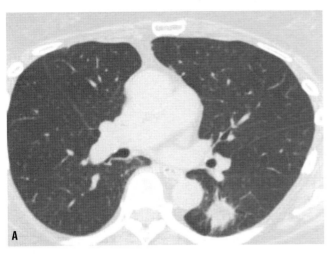

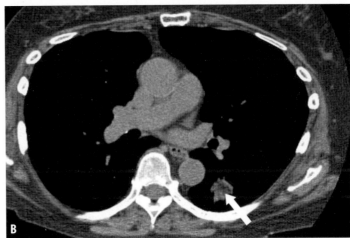

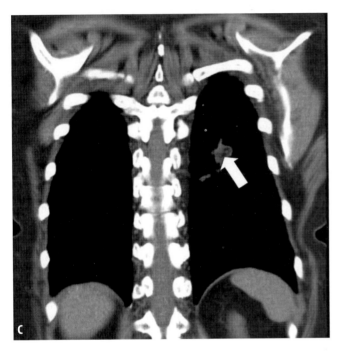

Figure 18.2 CT chest **A.** lung windows show an irregular mass-like area of consolidation in the left lower lobe. **B.** Soft tissue windows show fat attenuation (arrow) within the consolidation consistent with lipoid pneumonia. **C.** Coronal soft tissue window again shows the fat attenuation (arrow) of the consolidation. Patchy areas of lipoid pneumonia were present in other areas of the lungs as well (not shown).

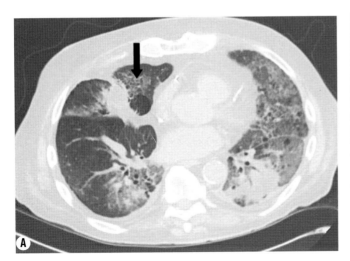

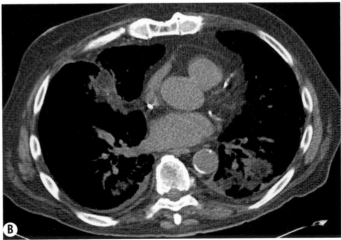

Figure 18.3 CT chest **A.** lung windows show bilateral areas of consolidation in the right middle and left lower lobes. There are also bilateral areas of ground-glass attenuation with some associated inter- and intralobular septal thickening (crazy-paving) (arrow). **B.** Soft tissue windows show fat attenuation in the areas of consolidation compatible with lipoid pneumonia. In this setting, the areas of ground-glass attenuation are also due to lipoid pneumonia.

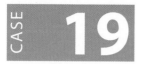
Pulmonary alveolar proteinosis

David Levin and Thomas Hartman

Imaging description

The classic appearance of pulmonary alveolar proteinosis is symmetric, predominately perihilar, ground-glass opacity with intralobular linear opacities and interlobular septal thickening ("crazy-paving" pattern) [1–3] (Figures 19.1–19.4). There is often geographic sparing of secondary lobules and periphery of the lung. Consolidation can be seen in advanced cases.

Importance

Pulmonary alveolar proteinosis is one of several conditions associated with a crazy-paving pattern on high-resolution CT. Knowledge of the different causes of this pattern can aid in preventing diagnostic errors [3].

Typical clinical scenario

Pulmonary alveolar proteinosis can have a range of clinical presentations. Most frequently it is characterized by an indolent and progressive course of cough, dyspnea, and sputum production [1–3]. The clinical symptoms are often less severe than the radiographic abnormalities would suggest.

Differential diagnosis

The classic "crazy-paving" appearance of pulmonary alveolar proteinosis is nonspecific. The differential diagnosis would include pneumocystic pneumonia, bronchioloalveolar carcinoma, pulmonary edema, pulmonary hemorrhage, nonspecific interstitial pneumonia, and lipoid pneumonia [3]. Although this pattern is nonspecific, differences in distribution as well as presence of additional imaging findings, together with the history and clinical presentation, can often be used to suggest the appropriate diagnosis.

Teaching point

In the clinical setting of indolent, progressive dyspnea, the crazy-paving pattern in a symmetric, predominately perihilar distribution should allow the diagnosis of alveolar proteinosis to be made.

REFERENCES

1. Holbert JM, Costello P, Li W, Hoffman RM, Rogers RM. CT features of pulmonary alveolar proteinosis. *AJR Am J Roentgenol* 2001; **176**(5): 1287–1294.

2. Chung MJ, Lee KS, Franquet T, et al. Metabolic lung disease: imaging and histopathologic findings. *Eur J Radiol* 2005; **54**(2): 233–245.

3. Rossi SE, Erasmus JJ, Volpacchio M, et al. "Crazy-paving" pattern at thin-section CT of the lungs: radiologic-pathologic overview. *Radiographics* 2003; **23**(6): 1509–1519.

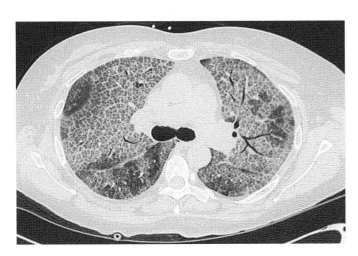

Figure 19.1 CT chest without contrast at the level of the carina shows bilateral symmetric, ground-glass opacities with a geographic distribution. There is interlobular septal thickening and intralobular linear opacities within the regions of ground-glass attenuation (crazy-paving pattern).

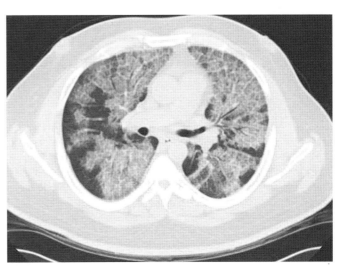

Figure 19.2 CT chest without contrast at the level of the bronchus intermedius shows bilateral symmetric, ground-glass opacities with a geographic distribution. There is interlobular septal thickening and intralobular linear opacities within the regions of ground-glass attenuation (crazy-paving pattern).

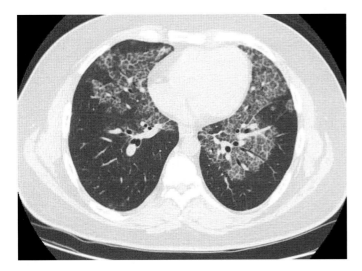

Figure 19.3 CT chest without contrast shows bilateral symmetric, ground-glass opacities with a geographic distribution. There is interlobular septal thickening and intralobular linear opacities within the regions of ground-glass attenuation (crazy-paving pattern).

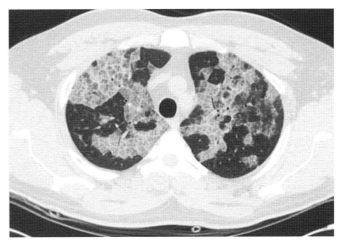

Figure 19.4 CT chest without contrast at the level of the confluence of the brachiocephalic veins shows bilateral symmetric, ground-glass opacities with a geographic distribution. There is interlobular septal thickening and intralobular linear opacities within the regions of ground-glass attenuation (crazy-paving pattern).

Alveolar microlithiasis

David Levin and Thomas Hartman

Imaging description

Alveolar microlithiasis is a rare disease of unknown etiology. Histologically, it is characterized by tiny calculi (microliths) in an intra-alveolar location [1, 2]. On CT imaging, innumerable tiny (1 mm) calcified centrilobular nodules can be seen throughout the lungs (Figures 20.1–20.4). The nodules tend to cluster in a perilymphatic distribution and can be seen on CT as high attenuation along the interlobular septa, bronchovascular bundles, and in the subpleural lung [1–3] (Figures 20.1–20.3). When the nodules are too small to be clearly identified as discrete nodules, they appear as areas of ground-glass attenuation in the lungs (Figures 20.2–20.4). When there is extensive microlithiasis, the calcifications can present as areas of "calcified" consolidation (Figure 20.1).

Importance

Although alveolar microlithiasis is a rare disease and individuals are typically asymptomatic, recognition of the characteristic findings allows exclusion of other potentially more significant diseases.

Typical clinical scenario

Individuals with alveolar microlithiasis are usually asymptomatic and the disease is typically discovered incidentally on a chest radiograph performed for other reasons [1].

If symptoms are present, it is typically dyspnea related to respiratory insufficiency.

Differential diagnosis

The differential includes other diseases that can result in pulmonary calcification such as metastatic pulmonary calcification and the diffuse interstitial form of amyloidosis. Metastatic pulmonary calcification is usually larger and has a more peripheral distribution. The diffuse interstitial form of amyloidosis can have interlobular septal thickening and ground-glass attenuation, however, it typically lacks the calcified centrilobular nodules.

> **Teaching point**
>
> Although a rare disease, the imaging findings of alveolar microlithiasis are typically diagnostic.

REFERENCES
1. Chung MJ, Lee KS, Franquet T, et al. Metabolic lung disease: imaging and histopathologic findings. *Eur J Radiol* 2005; **54**(2): 233–245.
2. Sumikawa H, Johkoh T, Tomiyama N, et al. Pulmonary alveolar microlithiasis: CT and pathologic findings in 10 patients. *Monaldi Arch Chest Dis* 2005; **63**(1): 59–64.
3. Cluzel P, Grenier P, Bernadac P, et al. Pulmonary alveolar microlithiasis: CT findings. *J Comput Assist Tomogr* 1991; **15**(6): 938–942.

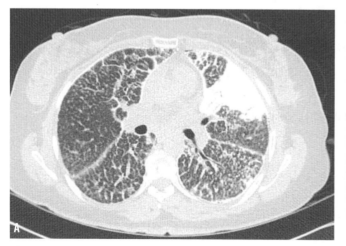
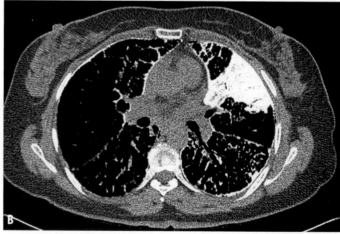

Figure 20.1 A. CT chest without contrast. Lung windows show centrilobular nodules and interlobular septal thickening bilaterally with an area of consolidation in the lingula. **B.** CT chest from same level as Figure 20.1A. Soft tissue windows show that the interlobular septal thickening and the consolidation are calcified. Note also the subpleural calcification.

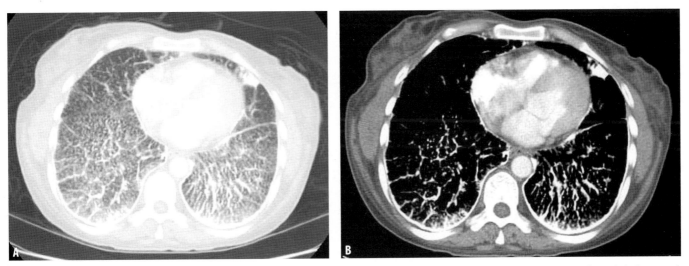

Figure 20.2 A. CT chest with contrast. Lung windows show centrilobular nodules, areas of ground-glass attenuation and interlobular septal thickening bilaterally with an area of consolidation in the lingula. **B.** CT chest from same level as Figure 20.2A. Soft tissue windows show that the interlobular septal thickening and the consolidation are calcified. Note also the subpleural calcification.

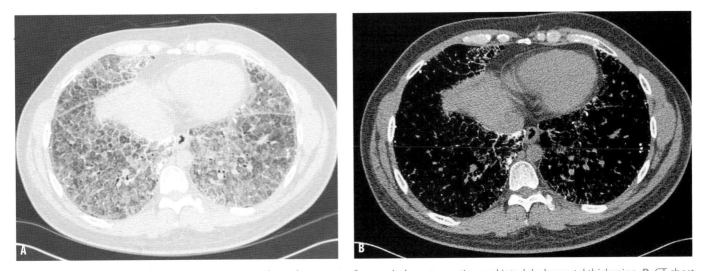

Figure 20.3 A. CT chest without contrast. Lung windows show areas of ground-glass attenuation and interlobular septal thickening. **B.** CT chest from same level as Figure 20.3A. Soft tissue windows show that some of the interlobular septal thickening is calcified.

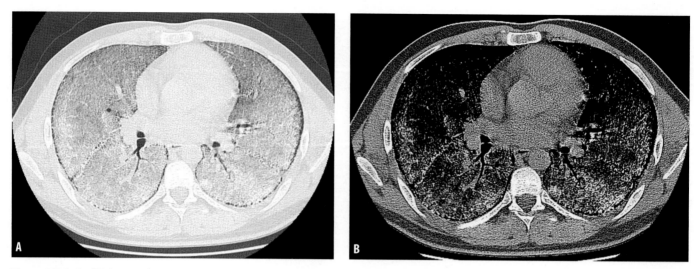

Figure 20.4 A. CT chest without contrast. Lung windows show dense ground-glass attenuation bilaterally that nearly obscures the underlying lung architecture. **B.** CT chest at same level as Figure 20.4A. Soft tissue windows show that the ground-glass attenuation is comprised of micronodular calcification.

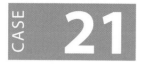
Metastatic pulmonary calcification

David Levin and Thomas Hartman

Imaging description

Metastatic pulmonary calcification on CT is characterized by patchy or confluent parenchymal opacities most commonly in the upper lungs. These are typically ground-glass, although there may be frank consolidation (Figures 21.1 and 21.2). The focal opacities often appear to be centrilobular (Figure 20.1) although histologically the calcium is located within the interlobular septa [1–3]. Punctate parenchymal calcification is a common feature (60%). There may also be associated calcification in the chest wall vessels. It is postulated that the lung apices are most frequently involved due to the relatively greater ventilation to perfusion and the relative tissue alkalinity [1–3].

Importance

Although metastatic pulmonary calcification is uncommon, the imaging findings can strongly suggest the diagnosis in the appropriate clinical context. If the diagnosis is uncertain based on CT, a nuclear medicine bone scan may confirm the diagnosis [4].

Typical clinical scenario

Metastatic pulmonary calcification is typically seen in association with chronic renal failure, hyperparathyroidism, and multiple myeloma. In these diseases, the high serum levels of calcium and phosphate lead to the deposition of calcium within tissues, including lung, kidney, and stomach. Regardless of the associated etiology, patients are typically asymptomatic, even when the amount of calcification is substantial.

Differential diagnosis

The imaging appearance can be similar to that seen with pulmonary alveolar microlithiasis. However, metastatic pulmonary calcification usually has an upper lung distribution while microlithiasis is diffuse. The clinical scenario can also help with the diagnosis. Other causes of pulmonary calcification such as dystrophic calcification or calcification associated with old varicella pneumonia have different imaging findings.

Teaching point

Metastatic pulmonary calcification is seen in diseases associated with high serum levels of calcium and phosphate. The pulmonary calcifications are characteristically seen in the upper lungs.

REFERENCES

1. Marchiori E, Franquet T, Gasparetto TD, Goncalves LP, Escuissato DL. Consolidation with diffuse or focal high attenuation – computed tomography findings. *J Thorac Imaging* 2008; **23**(4): 298–304.
2. Marchiori E, Souza AS Jr, Franquet T, et al. Diffuse high attenuation pulmonary abnormalities: a pattern-oriented diagnostic approach on high resolution CT. *AJR Am J Roentgenol* 2005; **184**: 273–282.
3. Marchiori E, Muller NL, Souza AS Jr, et al. Unusual manifestations of metastatic pulmonary calcification: high resolution CT and pathologic findings. *J Thorac Imaging* 2005; **20**: 66–70.
4. Rosenthal DI, Chandler HL, Azizi F, et al. Uptake of bone imaging agents by diffuse pulmonary metastatic calcification. *AJR Am J Roentgenol* 1977; **129**: 871–874.

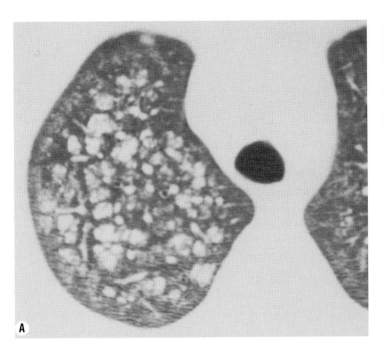
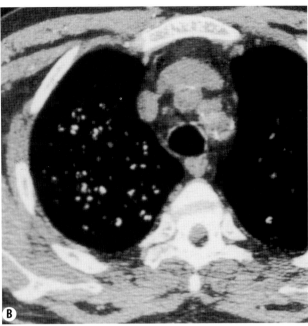

Figure 21.1 Targeted CT right apex in patient with chronic renal failure. **A.** Lung windows show ground-glass and more dense nodular opacities which mimic centrilobular distribution. **B.** Soft tissue windows show scattered calcifications in the nodular opacities in the right apex.

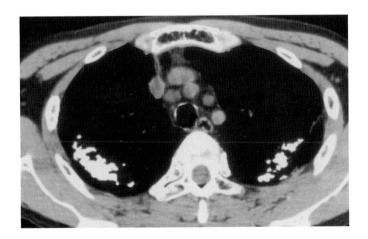

Figure 21.2 CT chest soft tissue windows show calcified "consolidation" in the lung apices in a patient with chronic renal failure.

Pulmonary hamartoma

Thomas Hartman

Imaging description

Pulmonary hamartomas are the most common benign tumor in the lungs. They present as solitary, round, well-circumscribed soft tissue opacities in the lung parenchyma on CT imaging [1–3]. Areas of fat (60%) or calcification (26%) can be seen within the nodule [1]. When areas of fat are identified in a nodule on CT imaging, the diagnosis of hamartoma can typically be made (Figures 22.1–22.3).

Importance

Hamartomas are benign lesions that do not need further workup or resection if they are asymptomatic. Since they usually present as an indeterminate nodule on the chest radiograph, a CT is often obtained to exclude malignancy. Recognition of fat within the nodule on CT will make the diagnosis of hamartoma and will exclude malignancy.

Typical clinical scenario

Hamartomas are almost always asymptomatic and discovered incidentally on a chest radiograph done for another indication [1–3]. In the rare instances when hamartomas cause symptoms, the symptoms are usually related to mass effect on adjacent structures such as airways or vessels [2].

Differential diagnosis

When fat is seen in a nodule on CT images, the diagnosis of hamartoma can usually be made with confidence. The other potential fat-containing nodule that may be seen would be a liposarcoma metastasis. However, clinical history would help in the differential and most liposarcoma metastases do not contain visible fat on CT.

When there is no fat seen on CT images, it is not possible to differentiate a hamartoma from nodules due to malignancy or infection based on imaging [1, 2].

Teaching point

A solitary pulmonary nodule that is shown to contain fat on CT imaging can be diagnosed as a hamartoma and does not need further workup or resection.

REFERENCES

1. Siegelman SS, Khouri NF, Scott WW, Jr, et al. Pulmonary hamartoma: CT findings. *Radiology* 1986; **160**: 313–317.

2. Hansen CP, Holtveg H, Francis D, et al. Pulmonary hamartoma. *J Thorac Cardiovasc Surg* 1992; **104**: 674–678.

3. Gaerte SC, Meyer CA, Winer-Muram HT, et al. Fat-containing lesions of the chest. *Radiographics* 2002; **22**: S61–S78.

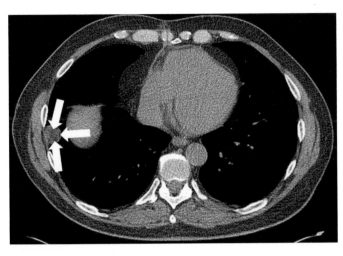

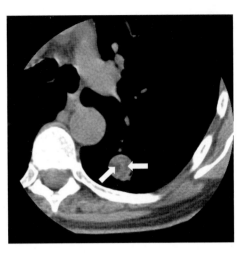

Figure 22.1 CT chest shows a large hamartoma in the right lower lobe laterally with visible areas of fat (arrows) within the nodule.

Figure 22.2 Targeted CT chest shows a hamartoma in the left lower lobe with visible areas of fat (arrows) within the nodule.

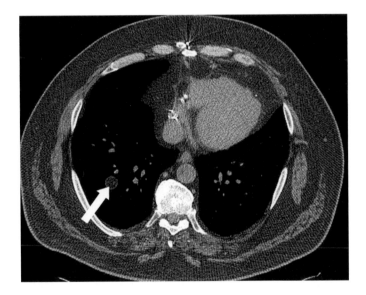

Figure 22.3 CT chest shows a hamartoma (arrow) in the right lower lobe that is almost completely fat attenuation with only a few small areas of soft tissue attenuation.

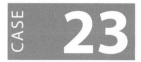

Carney's triad/pulmonary chondromas

Thomas Hartman

Imaging description

Carney's triad is characterized by pulmonary chondromas, gastrointestinal stromal cell tumors, and extra-adrenal paragangliomas [1]. As such, the primary imaging finding in the chest in a patient with Carney's triad will be pulmonary chondromas (Figures 23.1A and 23.2A) [1–3]. Occasionally, paragangliomas may also be seen in the mediastinum (Figure 23.2C) [1, 2]. The gastrointestinal stromal cell tumors may be visible on the lower images of a CT chest or can be searched for with an abdominal CT or MRI (Figures 23.1C and 23.2D). Pulmonary chondromas present as calcified nodules in the lung parenchyma. In chondromas, the calcification is chondroid calcification (Figures 23.1A and 23.1B), which can often be distinguished from other types of calcification by the "popcorn" appearance of the calcification [1–3]. In most cases of Carney's triad, multiple pulmonary chondromas are present.

Importance

Carney's triad is a rare disorder with only 79 cases reported in the literature [1]. It affects primarily young adults (<35 years) with 85% of cases occurring in women. Recognition of pulmonary chondromas should alert the radiologist to search the mediastinum and abdomen closely for associated paragangliomas and gastric tumors.

Typical clinical scenario

Pulmonary chondromas are almost always asymptomatic and are usually discovered incidentally on a chest radiograph done for another indication. Only two of the three legs of the triad have to be present to make the diagnosis and often the findings will occur at different times [1]. Therefore, some patients may have had prior diagnosis and resection of gastric tumors or paragangliomas before the recognition of pulmonary chondromas.

Differential diagnosis

Other causes of pulmonary nodules that can present with chondroid calcification should be considered. The most common of these is a hamartoma. When fat is present, in addition to the calcification, differentiation of the hamartoma is possible [3]. Also, hamartomas are almost always solitary while chondromas in Carney's triad are almost always multiple.

Metastatic lesions from a chondroid malignancy such as chondrosarcoma would be another consideration. The clinical history is often helpful in suggesting the possibility of metastases. Additionally, although chondrosarcoma metastases can be calcified, the majority present as soft tissue nodules without calcification.

Teaching point

When pulmonary chondromas are discovered on imaging of the chest, additional attention should be directed to the mediastinum and abdomen to look for associated paragangliomas and gastric tumors that allow the diagnosis of Carney's triad to be made.

REFERENCES

1. Carney JA. Gastric stromal sarcoma, pulmonary chondroma, and extra-adrenal paraganglioma (Carney triad): natural history, adrenocortical component, and possible familial occurrence. *Mayo Clin Proc* 1999; **74**: 543–552.
2. Marchiori E, Souza AS, Franquet T, Muller NL. Diffuse high-attenuation pulmonary abnormalities: a Pattern-oriented diagnostic approach on high-resolution CT. *AJR Am J Roentgenol* 2005; **184**(1): 273–282.
3. Bini A, Grazia M, Petrella F, Chittolini M. Multiple chondromatous hamartomas of the lung. *Interact Cardiovasc Thorac Surg* 2002; **1**(2): 78–80.

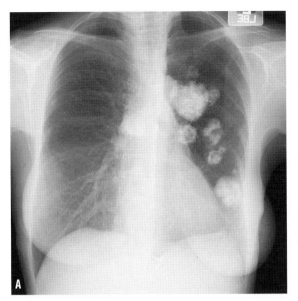

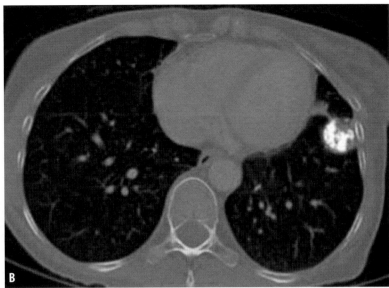

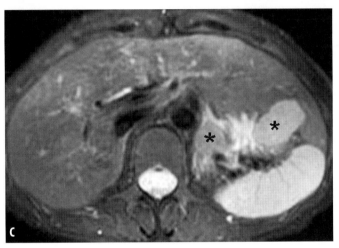

Figure 23.1 A. Chest radiograph from a woman with Carney's triad shows multiple pulmonary nodules and masses with chondroid calcification consistent with chondromas. **B.** CT chest bone windows showing chondroid calcification in one of the masses in the left lower lobe. **C.** Abdominal MRI shows two gastric masses (asterisks) that were shown to be gastrointestinal stromal cell tumors.

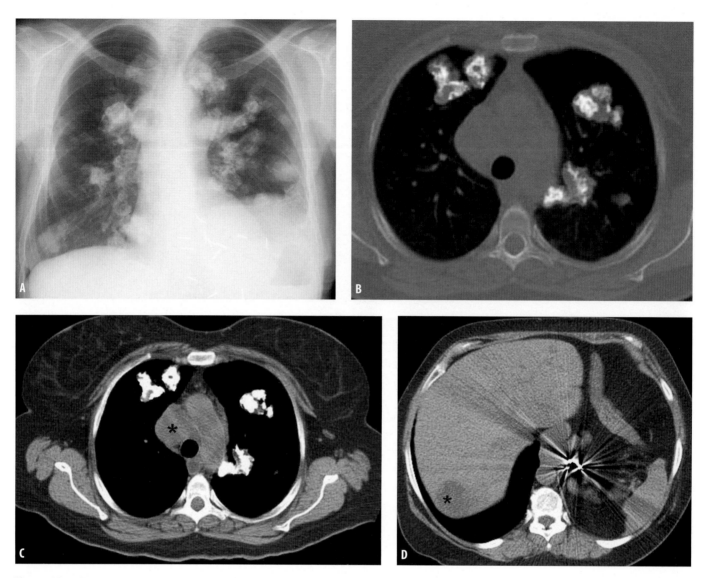

Figure 23.2 **A.** Chest radiograph from a woman with Carney's triad shows bilateral pulmonary chondromas. **B.** CT chest bone windows show multiple bilateral pulmonary chondromas. **C.** CT chest soft tissue windows show a large right paratracheal mass (asterisk) that was shown to be a paraganglioma. **D.** CT abdomen from the same patient as in Figure 23.2A shows postoperative changes of a gastrectomy and metastases in the liver (asterisk) from a prior gastrointestinal stromal cell tumor.

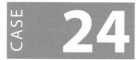

24 Mycobacterium avium-intracellulare complex (MAC) infection

Thomas Hartman

Imaging description

There are several ways that mycobacterium avium-intracellulare complex (MAC) infections can present in the chest. The classic appearance of MAC infection is indistinguishable from that of pulmonary tuberculosis. However, there is another presentation which has been called the "non-classical" pattern that is virtually diagnostic of MAC disease [1]. This pattern is a combination of nodules and bronchiectasis (Figures 24.1 and 24.2) and has also been termed Lady Windermere's syndrome. The nodules and bronchiectasis have a tendency to be more prominent in the right middle lobe and lingula, but can be seen in any part of the lungs [1–4]. Although the nodules and bronchiectasis are often present in the same lobes, they do not have to be in order to suggest the diagnosis. The nodules may be micronodules with a centrilobular distribution or can be larger with a more random distribution.

Importance

Infection with nontuberculous mycobacteria is an important cause of pulmonary disease. Of the nontuberculous mycobacteria, MAC is the most common pathogen. When the disease presents as nodules and bronchiectasis, the diagnosis can be suggested based on the imaging findings.

Typical clinical scenario

The nonclassical presentation of MAC disease is more common in women then men (4:1) and typically effects older adults. The most common symptom at presentation is cough which may be chronic [1, 2]. The disease is typically indolent, but on occasion can be progressive leading to respiratory failure and death secondary to lung destruction.

Differential diagnosis

Other atypical mycobacteria (kansasii, chelonei, etc.) are the most common infections to present with nodules and bronchiectasis, but on rare occasions other granulomatous infections such as *Aspergillus* and *Candida* can present with these findings [2]. Tuberculosis (TB) can also present with these findings although the apical distribution of the findings in TB is usually a distinguishing feature [3].

Teaching point

The findings of nodules and bronchiectasis with a predominance in the middle lobe and lingula in an older woman strongly suggests MAC pulmonary disease. However, since other atypical mycobacteria can have similar findings, it is more appropriate to describe the findings as compatible with atypical mycobacterial disease.

REFERENCES
1. Miller WT Jr. Spectrum of pulmonary non-tuberculous mycobacterial infection. *Radiology* 1994; **191**: 343–350.
2. Hartman TE, Swensen SJ, Williams DE. Mycobacterium avium-intracellulare complex: evaluation with CT. *Radiology* 1993; **187**: 23–26.
3. Swensen SJ, Hartman TE, Williams DE. Computed tomographic diagnosis of Mycobacterium avium-intracellulare complex in patients with bronchiectasis. *Chest* 1994; **105**: 49–52.
4. Primack SL, Logan PM, Hartman TE, Lee KS, Müller NL. Pulmonary tuberculosis and Mycobacterium avium-intracellulare: a comparison of CT findings. *Radiology* 1995; **194**: 413–417.

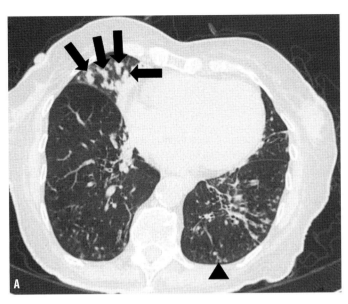
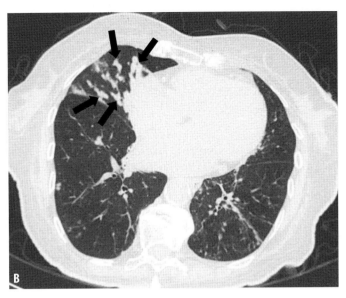

Figure 24.1 A. and **B.** CT chest in a woman with MAC pulmonary disease. Centrilobular nodules are seen in the lingula and both lower lobes with a centrilobular branching opacity in the left lower lobe posteriorly (arrowhead). There is bronchiectasis in the left lower lobe and right middle lobe. This is most marked in the right middle lobe where there is associated mucus plugging (arrows).

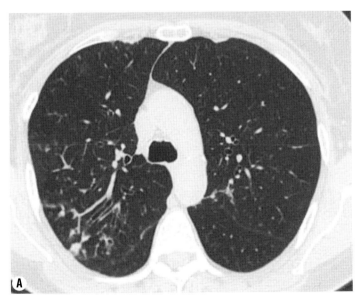
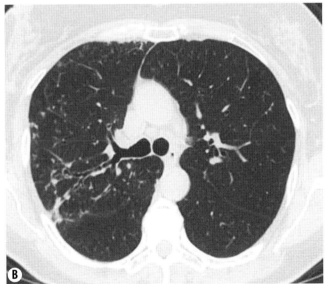

Figure 24.2 A. and **B.** CT chest in a woman with MAC pulmonary disease. Bronchiectasis in the right upper lobe posteriorly with nodules and micronodules in the right upper and left upper lobes. Additional nodules and bronchiectasis were present in the right middle lobe (not shown).

Mycetoma

Thomas Hartman

Imaging description

A mycetoma (fungus ball) is typically caused by *Aspergillus* superinfection of a pre-existing cavity or cyst. The mycetoma itself is characterized by a mobile soft tissue mass within a thick-walled cyst or cavity [1–3] (Figure 25.1). There is usually thickening of the pleura adjacent to the cavity. Common "cavities/cysts" that can be affected include those secondary to old granulomatous infections (tuberculosis, fungal), sarcoidosis (Figure 25.2), honeycombing in interstitial lung disease (Figure 25.3), bulla, and bronchiectasis from any cause. As such, the imaging findings in the lungs adjacent to or remote from the mycetoma may be influenced by the underlying disease. Mycetomas are usually solitary, but can be multiple and can occur in any location in the lung where a cyst/cavity has formed.

Importance

On the chest radiograph, a mycetoma may appear as a soft tissue mass in the lung and may be concerning for malignancy. However, the CT findings are usually diagnostic for mycetoma. Mycetomas typically have associated abnormal vascularity (bronchial artery hypertrophy) supplying the lesion and as such are predisposed to hemorrhage which can be significant. Approximately 10% of mycetomas will resolve spontaneously [1].

Typical clinical scenario

Mycetomas can be discovered incidentally on a chest radiograph obtained for another indication. When symptoms are present, they are most often cough and hemoptysis. Hemoptysis can be life threatening and may require resection of the mycetoma or embolization of the vessels supplying the cavity.

Differential diagnosis

The main differential considerations would be a region of necrotic lung or hemorrhage into a pre-existing cyst. Focal lung necrosis is most commonly seen in bone marrow transplant patients who develop invasive *Aspergillus* infections in the early post-transplant period [1, 3]. However, the specific clinical situation in the bone marrow transplant patient usually makes differentiation straightforward. Hemorrhage into a pre-existing cyst with clot formation can also mimic mycetomas [3, 4]. However, there is usually not thickening of the pleura adjacent to the cyst. Additionally, the clot will often resolve over a relatively short period of time.

Teaching point

Identification of a mobile soft tissue mass in a thick-walled cavity with associated pleural thickening should allow the diagnosis of mycetoma to be made. In the setting of hemoptysis, additional interrogation of the images may demonstrate the hypertrophied bronchial artery(ies) supplying the cavity.

REFERENCES

1. Franquet T, Müller NL, Giménez A, et al. Spectrum of pulmonary aspergillosis: histologic, clinical, and radiologic findings. *Radiographics* 2001; **21**: 825–837.
2. Logan PM, Müller NL. CT manifestations of pulmonary aspergillosis. *Crit Rev Diagn Imaging* 1996; **37**: 1–37.
3. Miller WT. Aspergillosis: a disease with many faces. *Semin Roentgenol* 1996; **31**: 52–66.
4. Knower MT, Kavanagh P, Chin R Jr. Intracavitary hematoma simulating mycetoma formation. *J Thorac Imaging* 2002; **17**: 84–88.

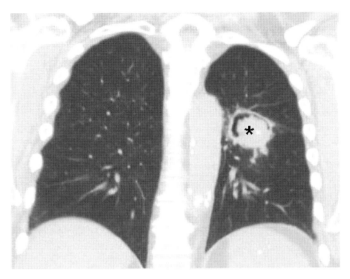

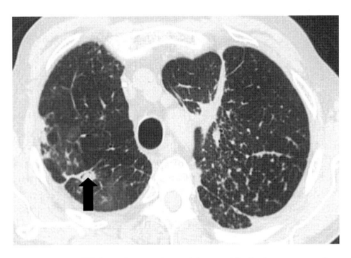

Figure 25.1 Coronal CT with lung windows shows a large soft tissue mass (asterisk) in a thick-walled cavity in the superior segment of the left lower lobe. Hemoptysis was the presenting symptom in this case.

Figure 25.2 CT chest in a patient with sarcoidosis shows a small fungus ball in the right lung (arrow).

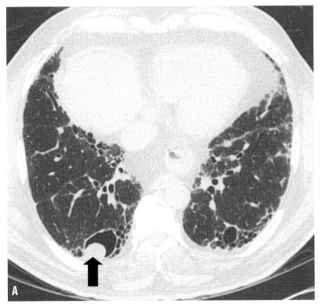

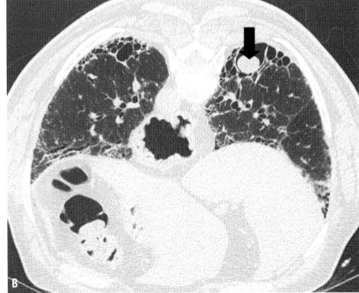

Figure 25.3 CT chest **A.** supine and **B.** prone in a patient with usual interstitial pneumonia and a mycetoma in an area of honeycombing in the right lower lobe posteriorly. Note the mobile nature of the mass on the supine and prone imaging (arrows).

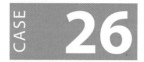

26 Rounded atelectasis

David Levin and Thomas Hartman

Imaging description

Rounded atelectasis has four key imaging features [1–3] (Figures 26.1 and 26.2). (1) The primary finding is a rounded, mass-like region of consolidation. Air-bronchograms are a common finding within the mass and the portion closest to the hilum typically has irregular margins. (2) The focus of rounded atelectasis should abut a pleural abnormality. Most commonly this is an area of pleural thickening. Pleural calcification can be seen. (3) There is a swirl of vessels and bronchi leading into the mass; the so-called "comet-tail sign." (4) There should be evidence of volume loss within the affected lobe commensurate to the size of the "mass."

Importance

Rounded atelectasis is a relatively frequent finding and the distinction from primary malignancy is important. When all four findings listed above are present the diagnosis can be made and no further workup is necessary.

Typical clinical scenario

Many patients with rounded atelectasis will have a history of asbestos exposure, typically with moderate and intermittent exposure. Rounded atelectasis can also occur following trauma and other causes of exudative pleural effusion. The mass-like focus is typically located within the lower lobes, lingula, and middle lobe. Most patients will be asymptomatic and rounded atelectasis will be an incidental finding.

Differential diagnosis

The primary differential consideration is lung carcinoma. Pneumonia is an additional consideration, although the clinical presentation is usually helpful in suggesting that diagnosis.

Teaching point

Rounded atelectasis is a relatively frequent finding and the distinction from primary malignancy is important. The identification of all four of the primary imaging findings is crucial to making the appropriate diagnosis.

REFERENCES

1. Doyle TC, Lawler GA. CT features of rounded atelectasis. *AJR Am J Roentgenol* 1984; **143**: 225–228.
2. McHugh K, Blaquiere RM. CT features of rounded atelectasis. *AJR Am J Roentgenol* 1989; **153**: 257–260.
3. Batra P, Brown K, Hayashi K, Mori M. Rounded atelectasis. *J Thorac Imaging* 1996; **11**(3): 187–197.

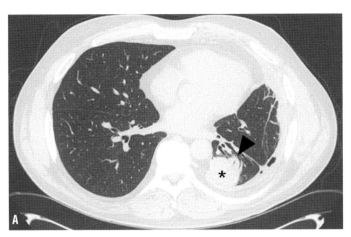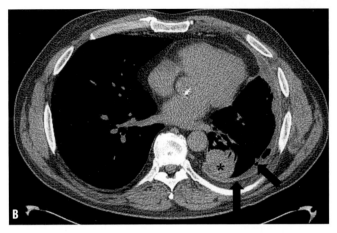

Figure 26.1 A. CT chest without contrast lung windows and **B.** soft tissue windows of an area of rounded atelectasis in the left lower lobe. Note the rounded "mass" (asterisk) abutting an area of pleural thickening and fluid (arrows). The "comet-tail" sign is seen anteriorly (arrowhead). Volume loss is indicated by the relatively posterior location of the major fissure.

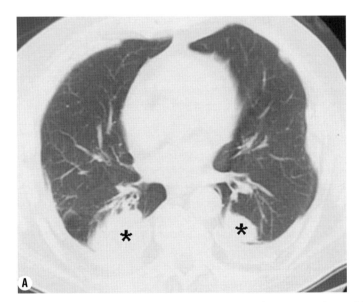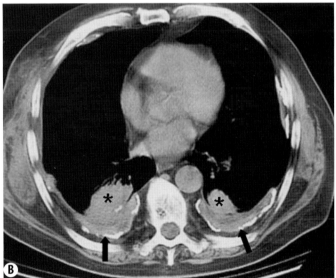

Figure 26.2 A. CT chest lung windows and **B.** soft tissue windows of bilateral lower lobe rounded atelectasis (asterisks). There are bilateral calcified pleural plaques from asbestos exposure (arrows).

27 Pneumomediastinum

John Hildebrandt

Imaging description

Imaging findings of pneumomediastinum consist of gas outlining the mediastinal structures (Figure 27.1). Gas within the mediastinum may dissect superiorly along the fascial planes, which can lead to subcutaneous emphysema in the neck and anterior chest (Figure 27.1). Occasionally the gas can dissect along the peribronchovascular interstitial tissue into the fissural pleura. A pneumothorax can occur from gas rupturing from the fissural pleura or directly from the mediastinal pleura. The gas can also extend between the heart and diaphragm giving the appearance of air along the entire diaphragm. This is known as the *continuous diaphragm sign* [1]. Gas in the mediastinum can also dissect to or from the abdomen via the retroperitoneal space (Figure 27.1).

Importance

It is important to know the etiology of a pneumomediastinum. Spontaneous pneumomediastinum generally has a benign course. However, potentially life-threatening complications such as tension pneumothorax or tension pneumomediastinum [2] can occur. Other serious causes of pneumomediastinum include perforation of the esophagus, trachea or bronchus, or hollow abdominal viscus. If pneumomediastinum persists or the etiology is unclear, further evaluation with CT abdomen, esophagram, esophagoscopy, or bronchoscopy may need to be performed.

Typical clinical scenario

Pneumomediastinum can occur spontaneously with a reported incidence of 1:800 to 1:42 000 [3]. These patients generally present with retrosternal chest pain, dyspnea, and occasional dysphagia. Mechanical ventilation, activities that result in a Valsalva maneuver such as retching or vomiting [4], coughing, sneezing, or childbirth are all reported causes of pneumomediastinum. Asthma and interstitial fibrosis are predisposing conditions to the development of pneumomediastinum.

Differential diagnosis

Air within the mediastinum is virtually diagnostic of pneumomediastinum, however, there may be some confusion with pneumopericardium. This can usually be easily differentiated since pneumomediastinum typically will have gas extending into structures remote from the pericardium and may have associated subcutaneous emphysema. Mediastinal gas can also be differentiated from pleural gas (pneumothorax) since the gas is confined to the mediastinum and does not surround the lung. However, it should be remembered that pneumomediastinum, pneumopericardium, and pneumothorax may coexist in a single patient.

> ### Teaching point
>
> It is important to identify the precipitating event causing the pneumomediastinum so as not to overlook serious abnormalities such as perforation of the esophagus, trachea, or hollow abdominal viscus.

REFERENCES

1. Levin DLL. The continuous diaphragm sign. A newly recognized sign of pneumomediastinum. *Clin Radiol* 1973; **24**: 337–338.
2. Macklin MT, Macklin CC. Malignant interstitial emphysema of the lungs and mediastinum has an important occult complication in many respiratory distresses and other conditions: an interpretation of the clinical literature in the light of laboratory experiment. *Medicine* 1944; **23**: 281–358.
3. NewcombAE, Clarke CP. Spontaneous pneumomediastinum: a benign curiosity or a significant problem? *Chest* 2005; **128**: 3298–3302.
4. Jougon JB, Ballester M, Delcambre S. Assessment of spontaneous mediastinum: experience of 12 patients. *Ann Thorac Surg* 2003; **75**: 1711–1714.

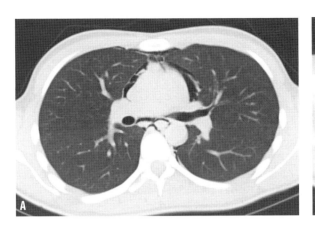

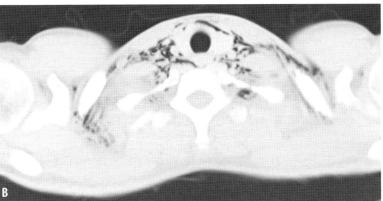

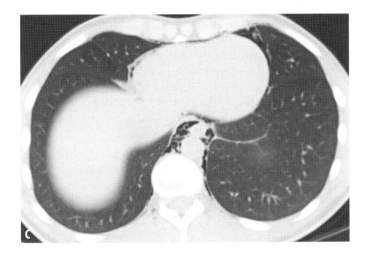

Figure 27.1 A. Axial CT demonstrates gas seen along the margin of the heart, esophagus, and descending aorta. The mediastinal pleural line is displaced away from the anterior chest wall. **B.** Axial CT demonstrates gas dissecting up into the lower neck and subcutaneous tissues of the chest wall. **C.** Gas is seen extending down along the esophagus and aorta and can extend down into the retroperitoneal space.

Fibrosing mediastinitis

John Hildebrandt

Imaging description

Fibrosing mediastinitis is a rare disorder which is caused by the buildup of collagenous and fibrous tissue within the mediastinum. It can present as either focal or diffuse mediastinal disease. The focal form will be seen as a hilar or mediastinal soft tissue mass and the diffuse form as mediastinal widening [1]. Infectious etiologies are associated with the focal form and present with calcified hilar and mediastinal nodes [1]. Granulomatous infections from *Histoplasma capsulatum* and *Mycobacterium tuberculosis* are the most common causes [2]. The diffuse form is usually associated with an idiopathic etiology and calcification is rarely seen. The accumulation of fibrotic tissue leads to compression of mediastinal structures such as the superior vena cava (SVC), pulmonary veins and arteries, central airways (trachea and main bronchi), and esophagus. Many of the clinical and radiographic manifestations are related to extrinsic compression of the central airways and vascular structures.

Airway obstruction causing lobar atelectasis or pneumonitis is common (Figure 28.1A). CT is excellent for demonstrating the presence of calcification (which can be extensive) within the hilar or mediastinal mass (Figure 28.1B) and the extent of soft tissue causing narrowing of mediastinal structures (Figure 28.1C). Parenchymal findings can occur from causes other than airway obstruction. Venous compression may cause pulmonary vein hypertension resulting in interstitial and alveolar edema (Figure 28.2A). Intravenous contrast is useful for assessing involvement of the SVC, pulmonary veins and arteries, and associated collateral vessels (Figure 28.2B).

On MRI, fibrosing mediastinitis has heterogeneous signal on T1-weighted images and low signal on T2-weighted images due to the presence of fibrotic tissue [3]. MRI is more useful than CT for the evaluation of vascular involvement, similar for the evaluation of the central airway, and less reliable for the identification of calcification. Other causes of fibrosing mediastinitis include sarcoidosis, autoimmune diseases, drugs (methysergide), and retroperitoneal fibrosis.

Importance

Fibrosing mediastinitis commonly causes compression of vital central mediastinal structures such as the SVC, pulmonary veins and arteries, central airways, and esophagus. The less common diffuse form can be very similar in presentation to lymphoma or bronchogenic carcinoma.

Typical clinical scenario

Clinical presentation usually is based on which structures are most significantly compressed. Patients may present with vague symptoms of pulmonary venous hypertension such as dyspnea and hemoptysis. More specific symptoms may come from compression of the airway such as cough and postobstructive pneumonia or compression of the SVC leading to SVC syndrome.

Differential diagnosis

Differential diagnosis includes lymphoma, bronchogenic carcinoma, metastatic carcinoma, and mediastinal sarcoma. The imaging findings in the focal form, clinical course, and tissue biopsies separate this diagnosis from the others.

Teaching point

Fibrosing mediastinitis can present as either focal or diffuse mediastinal disease. The focal form is more common and presents as a focal mass often with calcification that causes compression of adjacent vital structures, leading to clinical symptoms. The less common diffuse form has a similar appearance to lymphoma and bronchogenic carcinoma such as small cell.

REFERENCES

1. Sherrick AD, Brown LR, Harms GF, et al. The radiographic findings of fibrosing mediastinitis. *Chest* 1994; **106**(2): 484–489.

2. Mathisen DJ, Grillo HC. Clinical manifestation of mediastinal fibrosis and histoplasmosis. *Ann Thorac Surg* 1992; **54**(6): 1053–1057.

3. Rholl KS, Levitt RG, Glazer HC. Magnetic resonance imaging of fibrosing mediastinitis. *AJR Am J Roentgenol* 1985; **145**(2): 255–259.

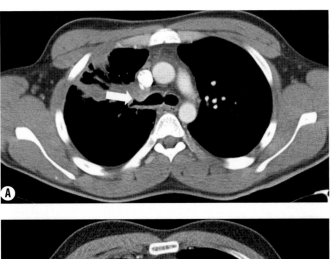

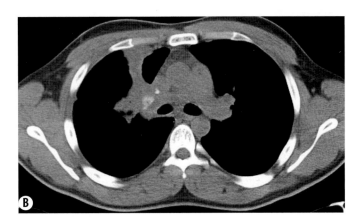

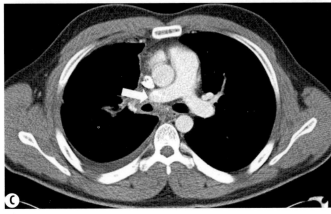

Figure 28.1 A. Contrast-enhanced axial CT chest demonstrates soft tissue narrowing of the right upper lobe bronchus (arrow) causing postobstructive atelectasis. **B.** Noncontrast axial CT image demonstrates calcification within right mediastinal soft tissue. **C.** Contrast-enhanced CT demonstrates right mediastinal soft tissue compressing and occluding the central right pulmonary artery (arrow).

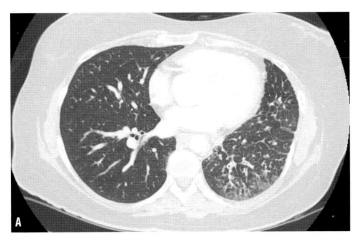

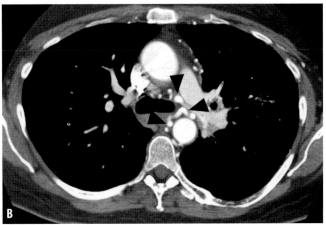

Figure 28.2 A. CT chest demonstrates interlobular septal thickening and mild ground-glass opacities due to pulmonary edema from occlusion of the left pulmonary veins by fibrosing mediastinitis. **B.** Contrast-enhanced CT chest demonstrates enlarged bronchial arteries (arrowheads) in a patient who had marked narrowing of the central branches of the left pulmonary artery.

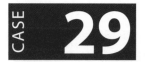

Extramedullary hematopoiesis

John Hildebrandt

Imaging description

On nonenhanced CT, extramedullary hematopoiesis (EMH) usually presents as a smoothly marginated homogeneous paraspinal soft tissue mass(es) in patients with chronic anemia [1]. The mass may contain fat, but soft tissue calcification or erosion of adjacent bone is absent [2]. On enhanced CT, the mass can have variable enhancement which is often inhomogeneous. The mass usually is heterogeneous on MRI and may have an increased T1 signal if fat is present [3]. Additional findings are related to chronic anemia and may include splenomegaly, coarse trabecular pattern of bone, and rib expansion (Figure 29.1). Extramedullary hematopoiesis can also involve the pleura and lung parenchyma [1] (Figure 29.2), and extrathoracic locations.

Importance

EMH is in the differential diagnosis of enhancing posterior mediastinal masses and can simulate neurogenic tumors, lymphoma, or pleural malignancy. There is a risk of bleeding with biopsy and rarely it can lead to spinal cord compression.

Typical clinical scenario

EMH occurs in patients with chronic anemia such as hereditary spherocytosis, thalassemia, sickle cell disease, and myelofibrosis. Patients are usually asymptomatic, but can rarely develop symptoms due to spinal cord compression [1].

Differential diagnosis

EMH is part of the posterior mediastinal paraspinal soft tissue mass differential and includes lymphoma, neurogenic tumors (paragangliomas, sympathetic ganglion tumors, nerve sheath tumors), and tumors of the pleura (mesothelioma, metastatic disease).

Teaching point

Extramedullary hematopoiesis is the likely diagnosis of bilateral posterior mediastinal paraspinal soft tissue masses in patients with chronic hemolytic anemia especially when there are signs of bone and/or spleen involvement.

REFERENCES

1. Koch CA, Li CY, Mesa RA, Tefferi A. Nonhepatosplenic extramedullary hematopoiesis: associated diseases, pathology, clinical course, and treatment. *Mayo Clin Proc* 2003; **78**(10): 1223–1233.
2. Yamato M, Fuhrman CR. Computed tomography of fatty replacement in extramedullary hematopoiesis. *J Comput Assist Tomogr* 1987; **11**(3): 541–542.
3. Savader SJ, Otero RR, Savader BL. MR imaging of intrathoracic extramedullary hematopoiesis. *J Comput Assist Tomogr* 1988; **12**(5): 878–880.

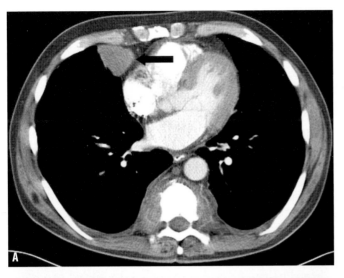

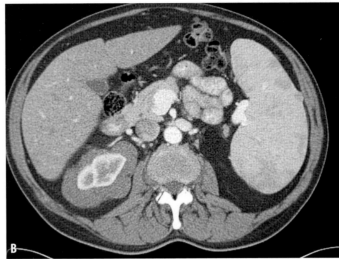

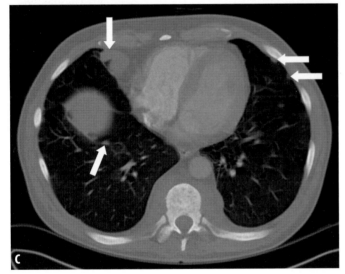

Figure 29.1 A. Axial enhanced CT chest in a man with myelofibrosis shows smoothly marginated paraspinal soft tissue and right anterior cardiophrenic pleural involvement (arrow) with EMH.
B. Splenomegaly secondary to myelofibrosis. EMH is also seen as the soft tissue mass surrounding the right kidney. **C.** CT shows sclerosis of the vertebral body secondary to myelofibrosis. In addition to the paravertebral soft tissue masses compatible with EMH, there are also pleural regions of EMH (arrows).

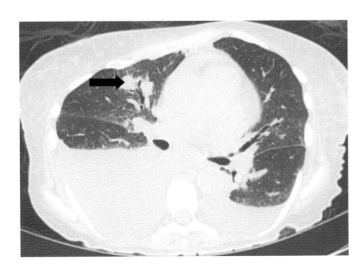

Figure 29.2 Axial CT in an 82-year-old female with biopsy-proven extramedullary hematopoiesis involving the pleural space and lung parenchyma (arrow).

Thymolipoma

John Hildebrandt

Imaging description

Thymolipomas consist of mature adipose tissue and normal thymic tissue. On CT, they present as a well-circumscribed, large fat density mass in the anterior mediastinum (Figure 30.1). They may extend down to the costophrenic angles as they become large [1, 2] (Figure 30.2). The soft tissue present is usually seen as linear bands between areas of fat, but can present as small round opacities [1, 2]. On MRI, the fat is seen as high signal intensity on T1-weighted images and the soft tissue as low to intermediate signal intensity [3]. In thymolipomas with large amounts of fat, the lesions tend to conform to the contours of adjacent structures without causing mass effect (Figure 30.2) [2]. Change of shape of thymolipomas can be seen with change in position because of the relatively "soft" nature of the lesion secondary to the prominent fat content [2].

Importance

Thymolipomas are benign tumors of the thymus that represent 2–10% of all thymic neoplasms [4]. They can be very large at the time of detection as they are slow growing and generally do not cause symptoms. However, in one study over 50% presented with symptoms including infection, chest pain, and dyspnea [2].

Typical clinical scenario

Large asymptomatic anterior mediastinal mass found incidentally on chest imaging at any age range with most diagnosed in young adulthood [1]. There is no sex predilection.

Because the lesions can conform to the adjacent mediastinal structures, the thymolipoma may be mistaken for cardiomegaly or elevation of the hemidiaphragm on the chest radiograph.

Differential diagnosis

The differential diagnosis includes other fat-containing mediastinal masses such as lipomas, liposarcomas, mediastinal fat pad, omental herniation, and mature teratoma. However, the lack of significant mass effect and the changing shape with change in position typically allow the diagnosis of thymolipoma to be made.

Teaching point

Thymolipomas are benign tumors of the thymus that contain fat and soft tissue and can be very large at diagnosis. They often conform to the contours of adjacent structures and can change shape with change in position.

REFERENCES

1. Casullo J, Palayew MJ, Lisbona A. General case of the day. Thymolipoma. *Radiographics* 1992; **12**: 1250–1254.
2. Rosado-de-Christianson ML, Pugatch RD, Moran CA, et al. Thymolipoma : analysis of 27 cases. *Radiology* 1994; **193**: 121–126.
3. Shirkhoda A, Chasen MH, Eftekhari F, Goldman AM, Decaro LF. MR imaging of mediastinal thymolipoma. *J Comput Assist Tomogr* 1987; **11**: 364–365.
4. Fraser RG, Muller NL, Coleman N, Pare PD. Masses situated predominantly in the anterior mediastinal compartment. In: Fraser RG, Muller NL, Coleman N, Pare PD, eds. *Diagnosis of Diseases of the Chest*, 4th edn. Philadelphia, PA: Saunders, 1999; 2880–2882.

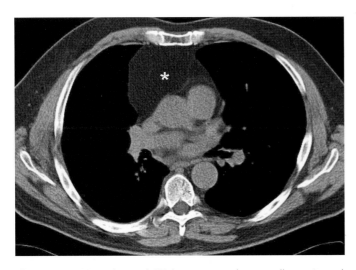

Figure 30.1 Nonenhanced CT demonstrates large, well-marginated, fatty, anterior mediastinal mass (asterisk) containing a thin central band of soft tissue.

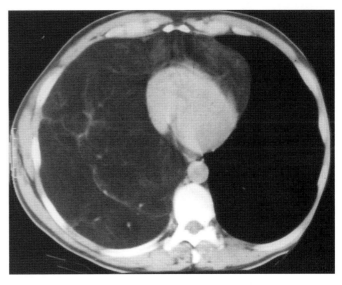

Figure 30.2 Nonenhanced CT chest shows a large predominately fatty lesion extending from the anterior mediastinum and filling the right inferior hemithorax. There are strands of soft tissue traversing the lesion.

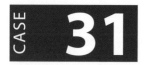

Mature teratoma

John Hildebrandt

Imaging description

Mature teratomas are made up of well-differentiated tissue from two or more embryonic germ cell layers. Thus, any combination of fat, fluid, soft tissue, or calcium may be present. In one large series soft tissue attenuation was observed in 100%, fluid in 88%, fat in 76%, and calcification in 53% of cases [1]. Although MRI is excellent at identifying various combinations of these tissues, CT is usually sufficient to make the diagnosis [1]. Lack of fat or calcification does not rule out the diagnosis, but the presence of these findings makes the imaging diagnosis more straightforward.

On CT, a mature teratoma presents as a well-marginated, lobulated, heterogeneous cystic mass with soft tissue in the form of septa or nodules along with components of fat and/or calcification (Figures 31.1 and 31.2). They are almost always in the anterior mediastinum. A fat/fluid level within the lesion is virtually diagnostic (Figure 31.2), but is reported to be present in only about 11% of cases [1–3]. Pure foci of fat or calcification may also be identified (Figure 31.1). The densities of the cysts on CT vary due to the amount of proteinaceous or lipid-rich material present. Thus the cystic components of the mass may also have a more variable appearance on MRI. Cystic components will vary from low to high signal intensity on T1, while soft tissue components are generally isointense to muscle and fat is high signal intensity on T1-weighted images (Figures 31.3A and 31.3B) [1, 4].

Importance

Germ cell tumors comprise about 10–15% of all anterior mediastinal masses. Of the various types of germ cell tumors, mature teratomas are the most common, representing 70% in children and 60% in adults [5].

Typical clinical scenario

Mediastinal mature teratomas usually are detected in children or young adults. In one series, the mean age was 24 years, and 83% were younger than 40 years old [1]. The incidence is similar in males and females. About half of the patients are asymptomatic at presentation [5]. Common symptoms include chest pain, dyspnea, and cough [5]. Uncommon symptoms may include pneumonia, hemoptysis, trichoptysis (expectoration of hair), superior vena cava syndrome, pleural and pericardial disease including tumor rupture into the pleural or pericardial cavities [1, 5].

Differential diagnosis

Mature teratomas are in the differential of anterior mediastinal masses. Differential includes hemangioma, lymphangioma, thymoma, liposarcoma, lymphoma, and thyroid tumors. The presence of multiple tissue elements such as fluid, fat, and calcification helps to differentiate mature teratomas from the other differential possibilities.

Teaching point

Combinations of multiple tissue elements within an anterior mediastinal mass suggests the diagnosis of mature teratoma. A fat/fluid level within the mass is specific although uncommon.

REFERENCES

1. Moeller KH, Rosado-de-Christenson ML, Templeton PA. Mediastinal mature teratoma: imaging features. *AJR Am J Roentgenol* 1997; **169**: 985–990.
2. Fulcher AS, Proto AV, Jolles H. Cystic teratoma of the mediastinum: demonstration of fat/fluid level. *AJR Am J Roentgenol* 1990; **154**: 259–260.
3. Seltzer SE, Herman PG, Sagel SS. Differential diagnosis of mediastinal fluid levels visualized on computed tomography. *J Comput Assist Tomogr* 1984; **8**: 244–246.
4. Ikezoe J, Takeuchi N, Johkoh T, et al. MRI of anterior mediastinal tumors. *Radiat Med* 1992; **10**: 176–183.
5. Hansell DM, Armstrong P, Lynch DA, McAdams HP. Mediastinal and hilar disorders. In: Hansell DM, Armstrong P, Lynch DA, McAdams HP. eds. *Imaging of Diseases of the Chest*, 4th edn. Philadelphia, PA: Elsevier Mosby, 2005; 921–922.

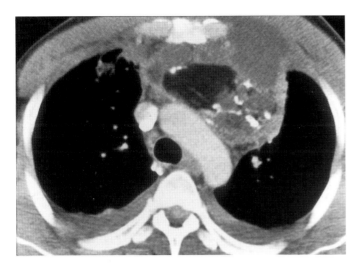

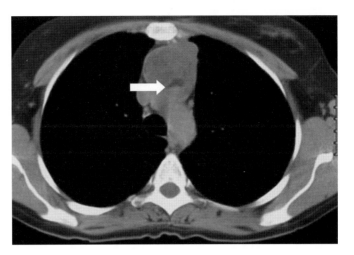

Figure 31.1 Contrast-enhanced CT shows a large anterior mediastinal mass containing areas of fat, calcification, fluid, and soft tissue compatible with a mature teratoma. Small bilateral pleural effusions are also present.

Figure 31.2 Nonenhanced CT of an anterior mediastinal cystic mature teratoma demonstrates a well-marginated, lobulated cystic mass containing a small fat/fluid (lipid-rich fluid floating over serous fluid) level (arrow).

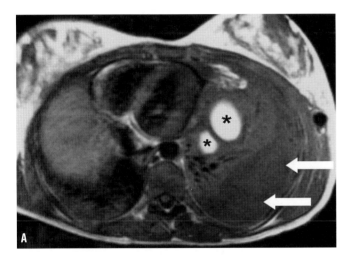

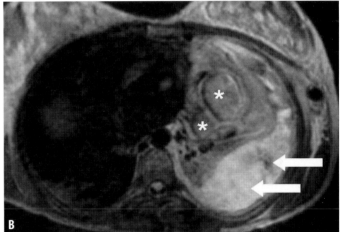

Figure 31.3 A. T1-weighted imaging, and **B.** T2-weighted imaging of a teratoma causing chest pain, recurrent pneumonias, and empyema. Left mediastinal mass contains high T1 and intermediate T2 signal of central cystic components (asterisks) due to high proteinaceous material, fat, or hemorrhage. Mass is causing atelectasis of the left lung, rightward shift of the heart, and a left empyema represented as high T2 and low T1 signal (arrows).

Mediastinal bronchogenic cyst

John Hildebrandt

Imaging description

Bronchogenic cysts most commonly occur in the mediastinum with the majority seen in the region of the tracheal carina [1, 2]. They can also occur in the lung parenchyma, pleura, and diaphragm [2]. On CT, a mediastinal bronchogenic cyst most commonly presents as a homogeneous fluid attenuation mass with a thin or imperceptible wall (Figures 32.1 and 32.2) [1, 2]. The attenuation of the cyst is influenced by the contents of the cyst and if there is a high protein content or calcium oxalate in the fluid, the attenuation values can be soft tissue or calcium [3]. Air is typically not seen in mediastinal bronchogenic cysts unless they are infected. The contents of the cyst do not enhance with contrast (Figure 32.1), but the wall of the cyst may enhance. MRI can be helpful in cases where the cystic nature of the mass is not apparent on CT. Although the signal intensity of T1-weighted imaging can vary due to the content of the cystic fluid, the cystic nature of the mass is confirmed by the high signal intensity on T2-weighted images (Figure 32.3) [1, 2].

Importance

Bronchogenic cysts are benign lesions. If they are asymptomatic, no further workup or resection is required. Therefore, identification of the cystic nature of the mass is important to prevent more aggressive intervention.

Typical clinical scenario

Most mediastinal bronchogenic cysts in adults are discovered incidentally during imaging for an unrelated cause. Symptoms are more commonly present in infants and are usually due to compression of adjacent structures by the cyst.

Symptoms can include chest pain, dyspnea, cough, and if the cyst becomes infected, fever and sputum.

Differential diagnosis

If the cystic nature of the mass is confirmed by imaging, the differential is limited to other cystic masses of the middle and posterior mediastinum such as duplication cysts, neurenteric cysts, and meningoceles. However, the location of the cyst and any associated spine changes usually help to differentiate the different lesions. If the bronchogenic cyst has higher attenuation on CT, then solid mediastinal masses may be in the differential. However, MRI can confirm the cystic nature and prevent misdiagnosis.

> ## Teaching point
>
> A cystic mediastinal mass with a thin or imperceptible wall in a subcarinal location should be a bronchogenic cyst and no further workup or therapy is required. In cases where the cystic nature is not apparent on CT, the high signal intensity on T2-weighted imaging should confirm the cystic nature.

REFERENCES
1. McAdams HP, Kirejczyk WM, Rosado-de-Christenson ML, Matsumoto S. Bronchogenic cyst: imaging features with clinical and histopathologic correlation. *Radiology* 2000; **217**: 441–446.
2. Jeung MY, Gasser B, Gangi A, et al. Imaging of cystic masses of the mediastinum. *Radiographics* 2002; **22**: S79–S93.
3. Mendelson DS, Rose JS, Efremidis SC, Kirschner PA, Cohen BA. Bronchogenic cysts with high CT numbers. *AJR Am J Roentgenol* 1983; **140**: 463–465.

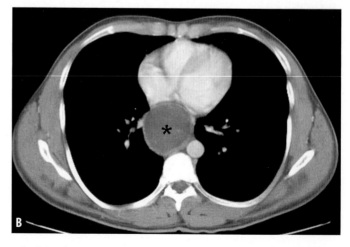

Figure 32.1 A. CT chest without contrast, and **B.** CT chest with contrast of a bronchogenic cyst (asterisk). Note the homogeneous fluid attenuation of the mass on both images. There is no enhancement of the mass with contrast although there is enhancement of a thin wall.

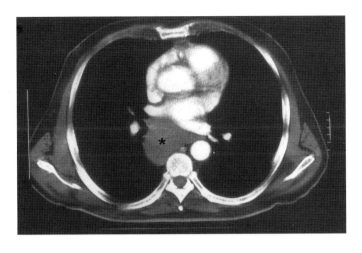

Figure 32.2 CT chest without contrast of a bronchogenic cyst (asterisk) shows a homogeneous fluid attenuation mass in the subcarinal region without a perceptible wall.

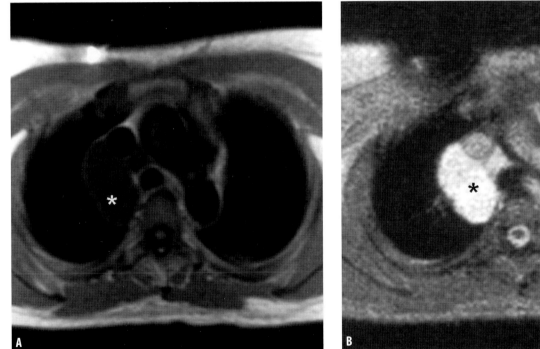

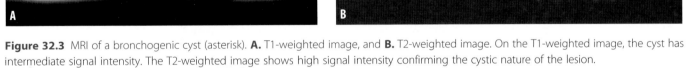

Figure 32.3 MRI of a bronchogenic cyst (asterisk). **A.** T1-weighted image, and **B.** T2-weighted image. On the T1-weighted image, the cyst has intermediate signal intensity. The T2-weighted image shows high signal intensity confirming the cystic nature of the lesion.

Lateral meningoceles

John Hildebrandt

Imaging description

Meningoceles develop from herniation of the leptomeninges through an intervertebral foramen. They can be congenital or can be secondary to trauma or surgery. The lesions usually are 2–3 cm in size but can be considerably larger [1]. The diagnosis is made on CT with intrathecal contrast or MRI by demonstrating fluid attenuation of the mass and continuity of cerebrospinal fluid (CSF) from the thecal sac with the paraspinal lesion [1] (Figures 33.1 and 33.2). If the lesion is not fluid attenuation, it is indistinguishable from other neurogenic tumors on CT without intrathecal contrast. The paraspinal component is sharply marginated and can cause pressure erosions of adjacent bones. Enlargement of the intervertebral foramen is common [2]. Associated findings may include kyphoscoliosis with vertebral and rib anomalies [3].

Importance

Approximately two-thirds of cases are associated with neurofibromatosis [2]. The appearance and association with neurofibromatosis is very similar to neurofibromas.

Typical clinical scenario

Approximately 75% of patients present between 30 and 60 years of age and are usually asymptomatic [2]. Thoracic lateral meningoceles can be followed clinically or radiographically. Surgical resection is indicated when symptoms are present [4].

Differential diagnosis

Lateral meningoceles are in the differential of posterior mediastinal masses. They most closely mimic neurogenic tumors, but often have fluid attenuation which can suggest the diagnosis. Demonstration of their continuity with the thecal sac via myelography or MRI is diagnostic.

Teaching point

Lateral meningoceles are benign lesions caused by herniation of the leptomeninges that contain CSF. They can be diagnosed by their imaging findings and only require treatment if symptoms develop.

REFERENCES

1. Strollo DC, Rosado-de-Christenson ML, Jett JR. Primary mediastinal tumors: part ll. Tumors of the middle and posterior mediastinum. *Chest* 1997; **112**: 1344–1357.
2. Miles J, Pennybacker J, Sheldon P. Intrathoracic meningocele: its development and association with neurofibromatosis. *J Neurol Neurosurg Psychiatry* 1969; **32**: 99–110.
3. Bourgouin PM, Shepard JO, Moore EH, McLoud TC. Plexiform neurofibromatosis of the mediastinum: CT appearance. *AJR Am J Roentgenol* 1988; **151**: 461–463.
4. Canvasser DA, Naunheim KS. Thoracoscopic management of posterior mediastinal tumors. *Chest Surg Clin N Am* 1996; **6**: 53–67.

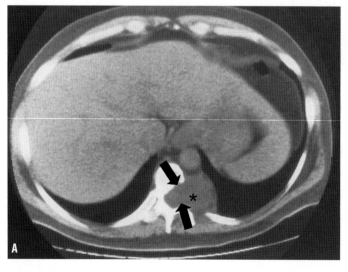
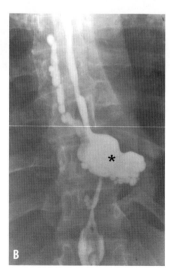

Figure 33.1 A. CT and **B.** myelogram of a lateral meningocele (asterisk) arising from the left lower thoracic spinal canal. Note the fluid attenuation of the lesion and expansion of the neural foramen (arrows) on the CT and the continuation of the lesion with the thecal sac on the myelogram.

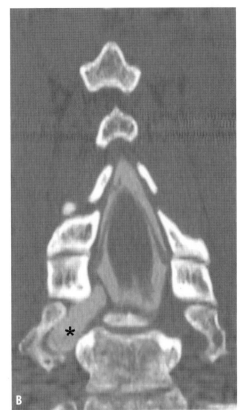

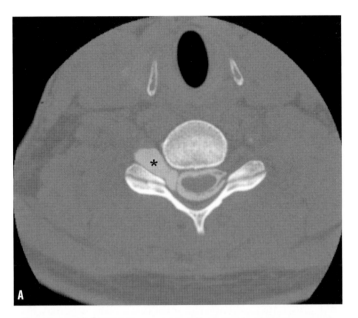

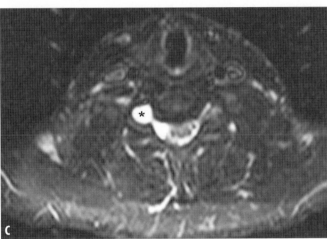

Figure 33.2 A. Axial and **B.** coronal CT with intrathecal contrast, and **C.** T2-weighted MRI of a small lateral meningocele at the right cervicothoracic junction (asterisk). CT with intrathecal contrast and T2 imaging demonstrates cerebrospinal fluid from the intrathecal sac extending out of the intervertebral foramen.

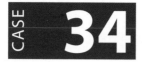

Peripheral nerve sheath tumors

John Hildebrandt

Imaging description

Mediastinal peripheral nerve sheath tumors (schwannoma and neurofibroma) almost always present as a paraspinal soft tissue mass in the posterior mediastinum. They have sharply defined margins and are round or lobulated in shape. Peripheral nerve sheath tumors generally follow the horizontal axis of the nerve. In 50% of cases, they apply pressure to adjacent bony structures leading to widening of the neural foramen or erosion of an adjacent rib or vertebral body (Figures 34.1 and 34.2) [1]. Ten percent extend through the adjacent intervertebral foramen into the spinal canal and form an "hourglass" or "dumbbell" shape (Figure 34.1) [1]. The mass has homogeneous or heterogeneous enhancement with intravenous contrast (Figure 34.1) [1, 2]. Punctate calcification is seen in 10% of schwannomas [3]. MRI findings include low to intermediate signal intensity on T1- and intermediate to high signal intensity on T2-weighted sequences (Figure 34.3) [4]. There is tumor enhancement with intravenous gadolinium (Figures 34.1 and 34.2).

Plexiform neurofibromas present as multiple paraspinal soft tissue masses which may extend along the ribs or into the anterior and middle mediastinum (Figure 34.3) [5].

Importance

Neurogenic tumors are common neoplasms of the mediastinum. They make up 75% of primary posterior mediastinal neoplasms. There is an association between neurofibromas and neurofibromatosis with 30–45% of patients with neurofibromas having neurofibromatosis [5].

Typical clinical scenario

Peripheral nerve sheath tumors are most common in adults [1]. Men and women are equally affected [1]. Schwannomas are the most common. Many do not cause symptoms and are discovered incidentally on chest imaging. Symptoms can occur and include pain or dyspnea from compression of intercostal nerves, the central airway, or superior vena cava [6]. Schwannomas and isolated neurofibromas have an excellent prognosis with complete excision.

Differential diagnosis

Solitary peripheral nerve sheath tumors are in the differential of posterior mediastinal masses. Differential includes neuroenteric cysts, tumors of the pleura, paraspinal abscess or hematoma, lateral meningocele, and esophageal duplication cyst. However, when a soft tissue mass causes expansion of the neural foramen, the diagnosis of a neurogenic tumor can be made.

Plexiform neurofibromas and extramedullary hematopoiesis can have similar paraspinal soft tissue findings. However, neurofibromatosis typically lacks the changes to the bones and spleen that are seen with extramedullary hematopoiesis. Also, in cases with neurofibromatosis, cutaneous neurofibromas may be seen.

Teaching point

Peripheral nerve sheath tumors make up the majority of posterior mediastinal tumors and a significant percentage of all mediastinal tumors. They are typically solitary lesions and when they expand the adjacent neural foramen the diagnosis can be suggested by imaging.

REFERENCES

1. Strollo DC, Rosado-de-Christenson ML, Jett JR. Primary mediastinal tumors: part ll. Tumors of the middle and posterior mediastinum. *Chest* 1997; **112**: 1344–1357.
2. Kumar AJ, Kuhajda FP, Martinez CR, et al. Computed tomography of extracranial nerve sheath tumors with pathological correlation. *J Comput Assist Tomogr* 1983; **7**: 857–865.
3. Ko SF, Lee TY, Lin JW, et al. Thoracic neurilemomas: an analysis of computed tomography findings in 36 patients. *J Thorac Imaging* 1998; **13**(1): 21–26.
4. Sakai F, Sone S, Kiyono K, et al. Intrathoracic neurogenic tumors: MR-pathologic correlation. *AJR Am J Roentgenol* 1992; **159**: 279–283.
5. Reed JC, Kagan-Hallett K, Feigin DS. Neural tumors of the thorax: subject review from the AFIP. *Radiology* 1978; **126**: 9–17.
6. Hoffman OA, Gillespie DJ, Aughenbaugh GL, Brown LR. Primary mediastinal neoplasms (other than thymoma). *Mayo Clin Proc* 1993; **68**(9): 880–891.

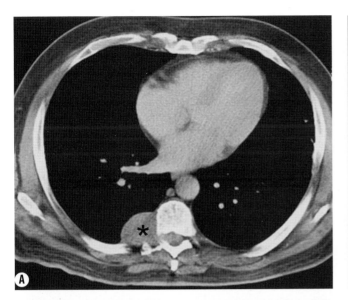

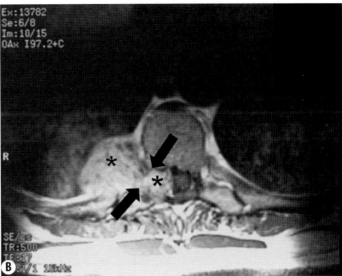

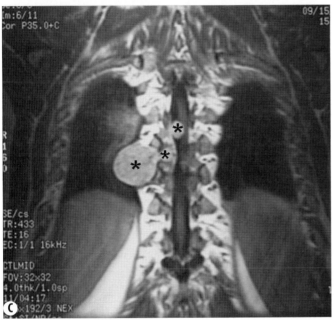

Figure 34.1 A. Contrast-enhanced CT and **B.** enhanced axial T1-weighted, and **C.** coronal T1-weighted imaging of a schwannoma (asterisk). CT demonstrates a homogeneous right paraspinal soft tissue mass which has an intradural and extradural component extending through the right T7 neural foramen. MRI demonstrates slight heterogeneous enhancement of the right paraspinal schwannoma at level of T7 neural foramen. The tumor slightly widens the neural foramen (arrows) and has a lobular component extending superiorly in the intradural space. This causes the "hour glass" or "dumbbell" shape that the tumor can display. The intradural component of the tumor causes some leftward displacement of the spinal cord.

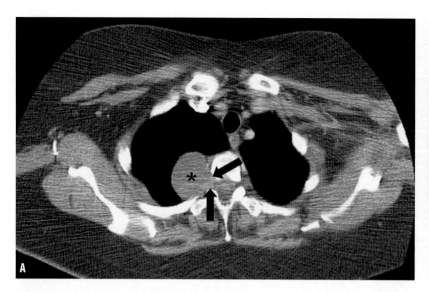 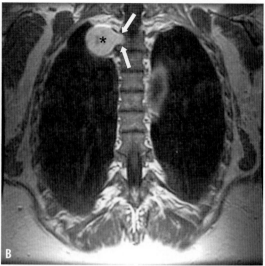

Figure 34.2 A. Unenhanced CT and **B.** coronal T1-weighted image of a schwannoma (asterisk). CT shows a homogeneous soft tissue mass which causes expansion of the neural foramen of T3 on the right (arrows). MRI shows a homogeneously enhancing lesion with a central scar causing expansion of the neural foramen (arrows).

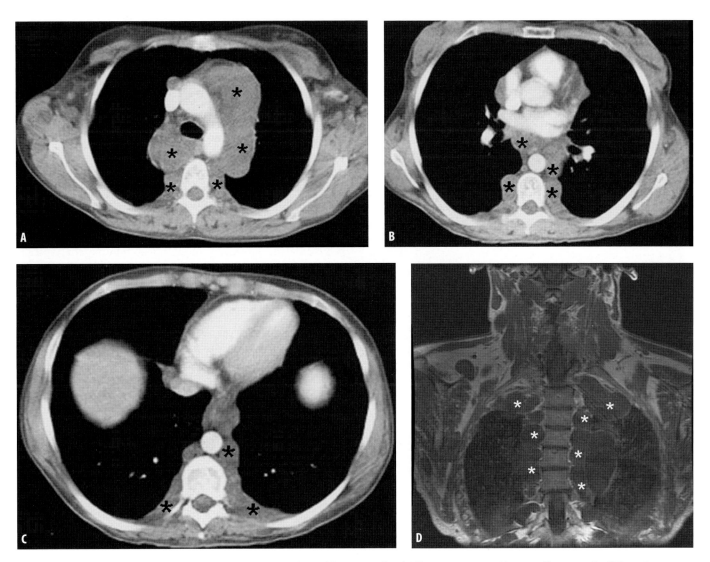

Figure 34.3 A.–C. Contrast-enhanced CT at multiple levels, and **D.** T1-weighted MRI in a woman with neurofibromatosis. CT imaging demonstrates extensive plexiform neurofibromas (asterisks) in a paraspinal location with extension laterally along the posterior chest wall and anteriorly to include the middle and anterior mediastinum. MRI shows homogeneous low T1 signal of paraspinal neurofibromas (asterisks).

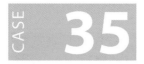

Fibrovascular polyp

John Barlow

Imaging description

Fibrovascular polyps are intraluminal masses that demonstrate mixed attenuation by CT. These pedunculated masses are usually smooth and sausage-shaped (Figure 35.1). They typically arise from the cervical esophagus. They extend inferiorly into the thoracic esophagus and can measure up to 25 cm in length. The diameter of a fibrovascular polyp is usually much greater than the diameter of the esophagus; consequently, these polyps distend the esophagus. Sometimes a longitudinal artery is demonstrated in the center of the polyp by CT with intravenous contrast material [1]. Esophagram confirms an intraluminal mass (Figure 35.2).

Importance

Fibrovascular polyps are rare, benign masses consisting of variable amounts of fibrous, vascular, and adipose tissue covered by normal squamous epithelium [2]. Imaging identification of fibrovascular polyps is important since up to 25% of these polyps are missed at endoscopy because they are covered with normal squamous epithelium [3]. Excision of fibrovascular polyps solves two significant problems: (1) progressive dysphagia and (2) the risk of airway obstruction and asphyxiation caused by regurgitation of the polyp into the pharynx [4]. Fibrovascular polyps do not undergo malignant degeneration.

Typical clinical scenario

Fibrovascular polyps cause progressive dysphagia. They may also cause weight loss and hematemesis. Polyp regurgitation into the pharynx can cause death by asphyxiation. In a review of 16 patients with fibrovascular polyps, one-fourth also reported "coughing, choking, wheezing, and/or inspiratory stridor" [2]. Esophagectomy is not indicated [5].

Endoscopic or surgical polypectomy relieves symptoms and prevents complications.

Differential diagnosis

The CT and esophagram findings of fibrovascular polyp are nearly pathognomonic. Sometimes intramural masses, such as leiomyoma, gastrointestinal stromal tumor, and carcinoma, may protrude into the esophageal lumen and even become pedunculated. However, these other tumors are typically more irregular, have a shorter stalk, and do not necessarily arise from the cervical esophagus.

> ### Teaching point
>
> Although rare, fibrovascular polyps have typical CT and esophagram findings. Polypectomy is performed to relieve dysphagia and remove the risk of asphyxiation secondary to polyp regurgitation.

REFERENCES

1. Kim TS, Song SY, Han J, et al. Giant fibrovascular polyp of the esophagus: CT findings. *Abdom Imaging* 2005; **30**: 653–655.
2. Levine MS, Buck JL, Pantongrag-Brown L, et al. Fibrovascular polyps of the esophagus: clinical, radiographic and pathologic findings in 16 patients. *AJR Am J Roentgenol* 1996; **166**: 781–787.
3. Ridge C, Geoghegan T, Govender P, et al. Giant esophageal fibrovascular polyp. *Eur Radiol* 2006; **16**: 764–766.
4. Carrick C, Collins KA, Lee CJ, et al. Sudden death due to asphyxia by esophageal polyp: two case reports and review of asphyxial deaths. *Am J Forensic Med Pathol* 2005; **26**: 275–281.
5. Solerior D, Gasparri G, Ruffini E, et al. Giant fibrovascular polyp of the esophagus. *Dis Esophagus* 2005; **18**: 410–412.

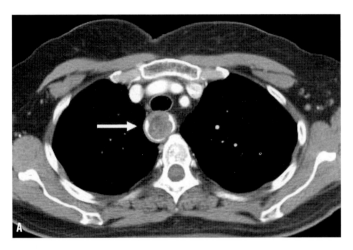

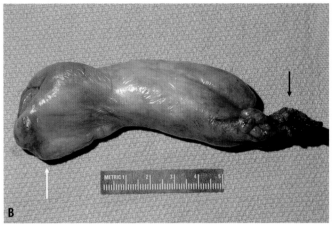

Figure 35.1 A. Axial image from CT chest with oral and intravenous contrast material in a female complaining of dysphagia, odynophagia, and weight loss. A large, mildly lobulated mass in the thoracic esophagus is nearly completely surrounded by esophageal contrast material (arrow). B. Gross photograph of the resected mass demonstrates its sausage shape, stalk (black arrow) and epithelial covering. The bulbous tip (white arrow) is a common finding.

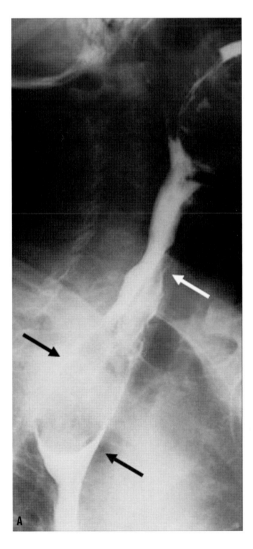

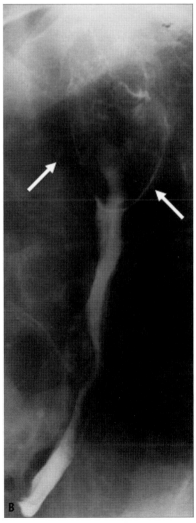

Figure 35.2 A. Upright left posterior oblique (LPO) view of the cervical and upper thoracic esophagus from single-contrast esophagram in a male with a mediastinal mass by posteroanterior and lateral views of the chest. The upper thoracic esophagus is expanded by a large, smooth mass (black arrows). The stalk, or pedicle, of the mass is demonstrated extending from the anterior wall of the cervical esophagus (white arrow). B. Prone right anterior oblique (RAO) view of the esophagus demonstrates a large, generally smooth mass that expands the proximal one-third of the esophagus (arrows).

36 Duplication cyst

John Barlow

Imaging description

A smoothly marginated, low-attenuation mass adjacent to the esophagus that does not enhance with intravenous contrast material is typically an esophageal duplication cyst (Figures 36.1 and 36.2). Sometimes the contents of these cysts are of intermediate or high density (Figure 36.3), making them more difficult to distinguish from solid masses [1]. Pre- and post-contrast-enhanced CT may be helpful to distinguish an intermediate density cyst from a solid mass. In cases that are indeterminate by CT, endoscopic ultrasound is the most direct means of distinguishing between solid and cystic masses of the esophageal wall [2, 3].

Importance

Esophageal duplication cysts are foregut malformation cysts. They are benign. The majority of duplication cysts are diagnosed in children.

Typical clinical scenario

Duplication cysts are usually asymptomatic and detected incidentally [4]. A large duplication cyst may cause dysphagia secondary to extrinsic compression of the esophagus. Some duplication cysts contain ectopic gastric mucosa; these cysts may be complicated by hemorrhage, infection, or rupture [1].

Differential diagnosis

Bronchogenic cysts may mimic duplication cysts; distinguishing them from duplication cysts is not important since they are both benign. The internal density of a duplication cyst is typically similar to fluid and, unlike a leiomyoma or gastrointestinal stromal tumor (GIST), does not enhance after intravenous contrast material administration. However, some cysts demonstrate higher internal attenuation because of protein or calcium oxalate or, less likely, hemorrhage or infection. Nevertheless, these cysts will not demonstrate internal enhancement after intravenous contrast material administration.

Teaching point

Duplication cysts are benign masses that are typically asymptomatic. Recognition of the fluid attenuation of the mass and the lack of contrast-enhancement can prevent confusion with solid esophageal masses that would require further workup. Occasionally, the attenuation of duplication cysts is much higher than fluid attenuation.

REFERENCES

1. Jeung MY, Gasser B, Gangi A, et al. Imaging of cystic masses of the mediastinum. *Radiographics* 2002; **22**: S79–S93.
2. Banner K, Helft S, Kadam J, et al. An unusual cause of dysphagia in a young woman: esophageal duplication cyst. *Gastrointest Endosc* 2008; **68**: 793–795.
3. Versleijen MWJ, Drenth JPH, Nagengast FM. A case of esophageal duplication cyst with a 13-year follow-up period. *Endoscopy* 2005; **37**: 870–872.
4. Naguchi T, Hashimoto T, Takeno S, et al. Laparoscopic resection of esophageal duplication cyst in an adult. *Dis Esophagus* 2003; **16**: 148–150.

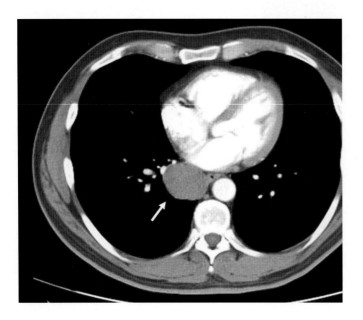

Figure 36.1 Axial image from CT chest with intravenous contrast material. A smoothly marginated right paraesophageal mass (arrow) is contiguous with the wall of the esophagus. The internal density of this mass is close to the density of simple fluid. These findings strongly suggest an esophageal duplication cyst.

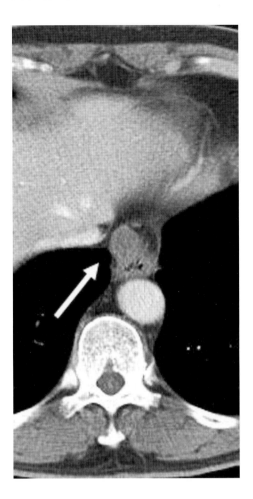

Figure 36.2 Axial image from CT chest, abdomen, and pelvis with intravenous contrast material in a male with lymphoma demonstrates a 2-cm oval, low-attenuation, well-circumscribed mass (arrow) contiguous with the anterior margin of the distal esophagus. This incidental finding, unrelated to lymphoma, should represent an esophageal duplication cyst. It had not changed since prior CT scan performed 10 months earlier.

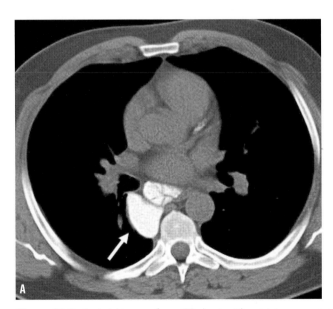
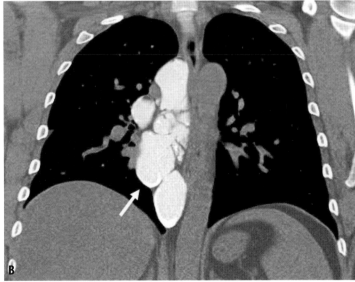

Figure 36.3 A. Axial image from CT chest without intravenous contrast material in a male demonstrates a multiloculated, high-attenuation mass (arrow) contiguous with the wall of the esophagus. B. Coronal image from CT chest without intravenous contrast material demonstrates the superoinferior extent of this multiloculated, high-attenuation middle and posterior mediastinal mass (arrow). Presumptive diagnosis is large esophageal duplication cyst or bronchogenic cyst. The internally increased density of the cyst should result from a mixture of mucus and protein or calcium oxalate.

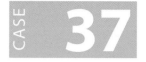

Pulsion (epiphrenic) diverticulum

John Barlow

Imaging description

A lower esophageal pulsion (epiphrenic) diverticulum contains some combination of air, fluid, and debris by CT chest. It may have an obvious connection to the esophagus because of a wide neck. The remainder of the esophagus may be distended since epiphrenic diverticula are caused by partial distal esophageal obstruction. Esophagram can confirm a suspected epiphrenic diverticulum by demonstration of a blind pouch, usually projecting to the right, connected to the distal esophagus by a neck. The diverticulum retains barium (Figure 37.1). Frequently, the esophagram also provides information regarding the functional or mechanical cause of partial distal esophageal obstruction.

Importance

Pulsion (epiphrenic) diverticula of the thoracic esophagus are less common than pulsion (Zenker) diverticula of the cervical esophagus [1]. Pathologically, a pulsion diverticulum forms when the mucosal and submucosal layers of the bowel are pushed through the muscular layers by increased intraluminal pressure. Pulsion diverticula of the thoracic esophagus typically arise distally secondary to increased intraluminal pressure caused by distal esophageal functional (motility disorder) or mechanical obstruction [2].

Typical clinical scenario

Epiphrenic diverticula are often asymptomatic – when symptoms are present they are usually dysphagia, regurgitation, or aspiration [3]. The evaluation of an epiphrenic diverticulum should answer two questions: (1) is the patient symptomatic? (2) Is a motor or mechanical cause of distal esophageal obstruction present? If both questions are answered affirmatively, diverticulectomy and relief of distal esophageal obstruction should be considered. When surgery is performed, diverticulectomy (Figure 37.1D) must be accompanied by relief of distal esophageal obstruction [2]. Epiphrenic diverticula may recur quickly if the distal esophageal obstruction is incompletely relieved [4].

Differential diagnosis

Epiphrenic diverticula can be distinguished from solid and cystic distal esophageal masses by their variable content of air, fluid, or debris by CT. Their appearance by esophagram is pathognomonic. The esophagram may also reveal the cause of partial distal esophageal obstruction.

> ## Teaching point
>
> When an epiphrenic diverticulum is suspected by CT, the esophagus should be further evaluated by esophagram or endoscopy – if these studies have not already been performed.

REFERENCES

1. Weitzman G, Maltz C. Epiphrenic diverticulum. *Endoscopy* 2006; **38**: E11.
2. Reznik SI, Rice TW, Murthy SC, et al. Assessment of a pathophysiology-directed treatment for symptomatic epiphrenic diverticulum. *Dis Esophagus* 2007; **20**: 320–327.
3. Fasano NC, Levine MS, Rubesin SE, et al. Epiphrenic diverticulum: clinical and radiographic findings in 27 patients. *Dysphagia* 2003; **18**: 9–15.
4. Valentini M, Pera M, Vidal O, et al. Incomplete esophageal myotomy and early recurrence of an epiphrenic diverticulum. *Dis Esophagus* 2005 **18**: 64–66.

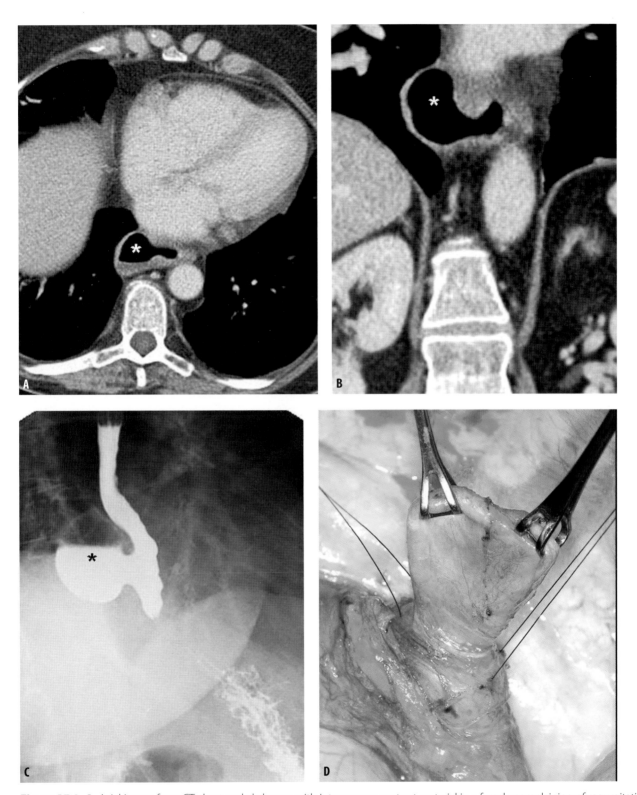

Figure 37.1 **A.** Axial image from CT chest and abdomen with intravenous contrast material in a female complaining of regurgitation. A saccular out-pouching protrudes to the right from the distal esophagus (asterisk). **B.** Coronal image demonstrates the thin wall and wide neck of the diverticulum (asterisk); it also demonstrates the proximity of this diverticulum to the diaphragm and the gastroesophageal junction. **C.** Upright left posterior oblique view from esophagram demonstrates the diverticulum (asterisk). **D.** Intraoperative photograph demonstrates the epiphrenic diverticulum under traction prior to resection. Distal esophageal myotomy was also performed to relieve functional obstruction.

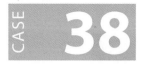

38 Traction diverticulum

John Barlow

Imaging description

By CT a traction diverticulum has the nonspecific appearance of a paraesophageal barium, air, or fluid collection. Traction diverticula typically arise from the mid esophagus, at the level of the carina, in association with calcified mediastinal lymph nodes (Figure 38.1). Unlike typically rounded pulsion diverticula, traction diverticula are often triangular [1].

Importance

Diverticula of the thoracic esophagus are classified by their location and their etiology [2]. Traction diverticula typically arise in the mid esophagus. A traction diverticulum includes the mucosal, submucosal, and muscular layers of the esophagus; it results from the pull (traction) of an adjacent mediastinal scar, such as those resulting from granulomatous infection. Traction diverticula are less common than pulsion diverticula of the distal esophagus that form when the mucosal and submucosal layers of the esophagus protrude through a muscular defect.

Typical clinical scenario

Small esophageal traction diverticula are usually asymptomatic. Larger diverticula can cause dysphagia and regurgitation. These large, symptomatic traction diverticula usually require surgical resection. Rare complications of traction diverticula include rupture and esophagobronchial fistula [2].

Differential diagnosis

The CT findings of a small traction diverticulum are similar to those of a mid-esophageal ulcer, contained rupture, and esophagobronchial fistula. Since most traction diverticula are small, barium esophagram or endoscopy is typically performed to differentiate between the etiologies.

Teaching point

Small traction diverticula of the mid esophagus are usually incidental, asymptomatic findings. If patient symptoms are suspicious for esophageal ulcer, traction diverticulum rupture, or esophagobronchial fistula, further evaluation of the esophagus by barium esophagram or endoscopy is indicated.

REFERENCES

1. Levine MS, Rubesin SE. Diseases of the esophagus: diagnosis with esophagography. *Radiology* 2005; **237**: 414–427.
2. Avisar E, Luketich JD. Adenocarcinoma in a mid-esophageal diverticulum. *Ann Thorac Surg* 2000; **69**: 288–289.

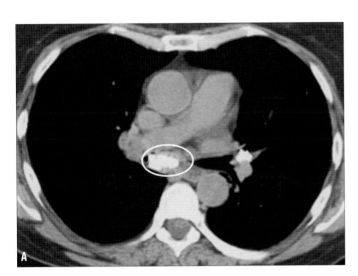
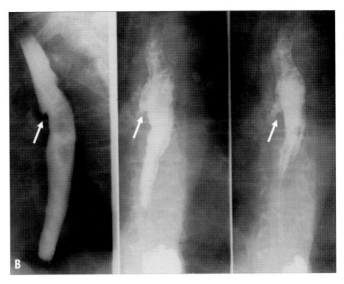

Figure 38.1 A. Axial image from CT without intravenous contrast material in a female complaining of cough while eating. Calcified lymph nodes are contiguous with the esophageal wall, but a traction diverticulum cannot be confirmed (white oval). **B.** Two upright frontal single-contrast views (right and middle images) and one prone right anterior oblique view (left image) from esophagram performed to exclude an esophagobronchial fistula. A shallow traction diverticulum protrudes from the esophagus (arrows) toward calcified mediastinal lymph nodes. A fistula was not confirmed.

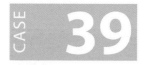

Esophageal downhill varices

John Barlow

Imaging description

Mid and upper esophageal (downhill) varices cause nonspecific thickening of the esophageal wall by CT chest without intravenous contrast material. These varices enhance after intravenous contrast material administration. Periesophageal varices are often present as well. Downhill varices are diagnosed by their location and by the associated signs of superior vena cava (SVC) obstruction (Figure 39.1). They are often smaller than distal esophageal uphill varices.

Importance

Downhill esophageal varices result from SVC obstruction; they are much less common than uphill varices secondary to cirrhosis and portal venous hypertension. Obstruction of the SVC often results from thrombosis and a common cause of SVC thrombosis is chronic catheterization. Other causes of SVC obstruction are mediastinal metastases, lymphoma, substernal goiter, mediastinal radiation, and sclerosing mediastinitis [1]. Blood bypasses the obstructed SVC by flowing inferiorly through esophageal and periesophageal veins into the inferior vena cava or into the portal circulation. Downhill varices are only one of many collateral pathways that blood can follow to return to the heart when the SVC is occluded; azygos, hemiazygos, and chest wall veins provide other collateral pathways. Therefore, the volume of blood flowing through downhill varices is typically less than the volume of blood flowing through uphill varices. Consequently, downhill varices tend to be smaller than uphill varices and are less likely to bleed than uphill varices.

Typical clinical scenario

Most patients present with SVC syndrome, secondary to SVC obstruction, before their downhill varices are discovered [1]. This syndrome includes venous distention and edema of the face, neck, and upper extremities [2]. Relief of SVC obstruction is the definitive therapy for downhill varices [3]. SVC obstruction is typically relieved by venous angioplasty (with or without stenting) or surgical bypass (such as internal jugular vein to right atrial appendage). When downhill varices bleed, they are often treated emergently with endoscopic banding or sclerotherapy.

Differential diagnosis

Downhill esophageal varices typically occur in a specific clinical context (SVC syndrome) and in association with specific CT chest findings (SVC obstruction). Consequently, no significant differential diagnosis exists when CT is performed with intravenous contrast material. However, these varices cause nonspecific esophageal wall thickening by CT chest without intravenous contrast material.

Teaching point

When SVC obstruction is diagnosed by CT chest with intravenous contrast material, evaluation of the upper and mid esophagus for downhill varices is warranted since these varices may bleed and a bleeding downhill varix can be a life-threatening situation.

REFERENCES

1. Levine MS, Rubesin SE. Diseases of the esophagus: diagnosis with esophagography. *Radiology* 2005; **237**: 414–427.
2. Cheng S. Superior vena cava syndrome: a contemporary review of a historic disease. *Cardiol Rev* 2009; **17**: 16–23.
3. Froilan C, Adan L, Suarez JM, et al. Therapeutic approach to "downhill" varices bleeding. *Gastrointest Endosc* 2008; **68**: 1010–1012.

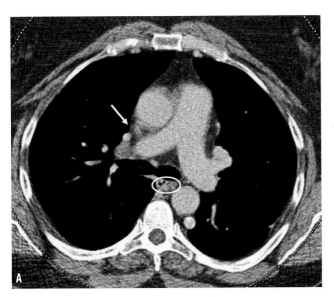 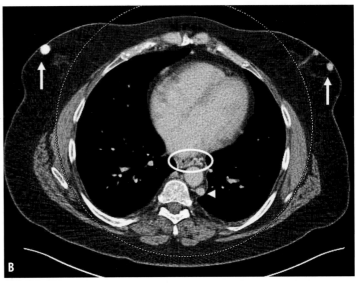

Figure 39.1 A. Dual energy CT chest with simultaneous bilateral antecubital vein injections in a female with SVC obstruction secondary to damage from chronic central venous catheterization. Periesophageal varices are demonstrated at the level of the tracheal carina (oval). The SVC is very small (arrow); more inferiorly, it was completely occluded. B. More inferior image demonstrates continuation of periesophageal downhill varices (oval). Large subcutaneous collateral veins are also demonstrated in both breasts (arrows). The hemiazygos vein is enlarged (arrowhead) by retrograde flow originating from a collateral connection between the left subclavian vein and the hemiazygos vein.

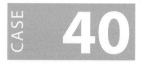

Esophageal uphill varices

John Barlow

Imaging description

Esophageal varices cause nonspecific thickening of the esophageal wall by CT without intravenous contrast material. After intravenous contrast material administration, varices enhance unless images are obtained very soon after contrast injection. As esophageal varices enlarge they become tortuous, tubular, and longitudinal (serpiginous) masses within the wall that cause lobulation of the esophageal lumen (Figures 40.1 and 40.2). They may be more prominent on the right side due to the presence of the descending aorta on the left. Esophageal uphill varices are often associated with CT findings of hepatic cirrhosis, splenomegaly, and gastric varices in the upper abdomen. Large varices have a higher risk of variceal hemorrhage. A conservative criterion for a large varix is a short-axis diameter of 3 mm or greater [1]. Paraesophageal varices are often associated with esophageal varices (Figure 40.3).

Importance

Distal esophageal varices in the setting of hepatic cirrhosis represent portosystemic venous shunts that form in response to hepatic fibrosis and increased portal vein pressure. They are sometimes referred to as uphill varices because they carry blood upward from the coronary veins of the stomach to the azygos veins. Distal esophageal varices are prone to hemorrhage. Variceal hemorrhage is a significant complication that carries a 6-week mortality of 11–20% [2]. Paraesophageal varices are not prone to hemorrhage.

Typical clinical scenario

Hepatic cirrhosis leads to portal venous hypertension that causes portosystemic shunts, including lower esophageal varices. Variceal hemorrhage is a significant cause of morbidity and mortality in cirrhotic patients. Beta-blockers are administered to patients with medium or large varices for prevention of first variceal hemorrhage [3]. Pharmacologic agents, endoscopic sclerotherapy and band ligation, balloon tamponade, transjugular intrahepatic portosystemic shunt (TIPS), and surgical shunts are all employed in the treatment of bleeding esophageal varices [4].

Differential diagnosis

By CT chest without intravenous contrast material, esophageal varices may cause nonspecific distal esophageal mural thickening that can also have infectious, inflammatory, and neoplastic causes. By CT chest with intravenous contrast material, varices typically appear as serpiginous masses that impinge on the esophageal lumen. The presence of hepatic cirrhosis and other signs of portal venous hypertension in the upper abdomen confirm the diagnosis of esophageal uphill varices.

Teaching point

When upper abdominal findings by CT chest suggest cirrhosis and portal venous hypertension, a search for esophageal varices is warranted. Estimation of the size of these varices is helpful in classifying the risk of variceal hemorrhage, a potentially fatal complication of portal venous hypertension.

REFERENCES

1. Kim YJ, Raman SS, Yu NC, et al. Esophageal varices in cirrhotic patients: evaluation with liver CT. *AJR Am J Roentgenol* 2007; **188**: 139–144.
2. Sharara AI, Rockey DC. Gastroesophageal variceal hemorrhage. *N Engl J Med* 2001; **345**: 669–681.
3. Garcia-Tsao G. Portal hypertension. *Curr Opin Gastroenterol* 2006; **22**: 254–262.
4. deFranchis R, Dell'Era A. Diagnosis and therapy of esophageal vascular disorders. *Curr Opin Gastroenterol* 2007; **23**: 422–427.

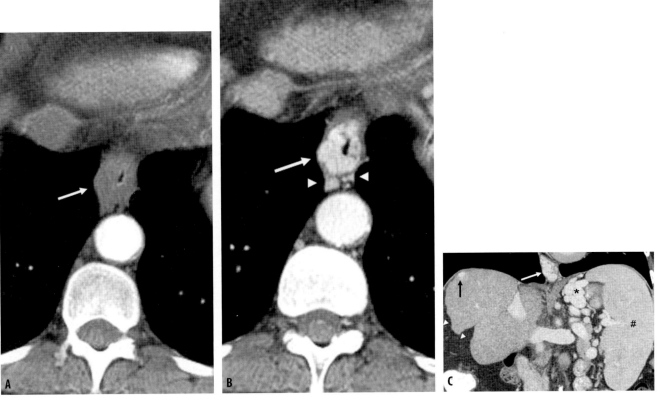

Figure 40.1 A. Axial CT chest and abdomen with intravenous contrast material (early arterial phase) in a female with alcoholic cirrhosis. Distal esophageal wall is thickened (arrow), a nonspecific finding. **B.** Late arterial phase images confirm that distal esophageal mural thickening results from varices (arrow). Small paraesophageal varices are demonstrated posteriorly (arrowheads). **C.** Coronal reconstruction of the lower chest and upper abdomen demonstrates irregular margins (white arrowheads) of cirrhotic liver, presumed small hepatocellular carcinoma (black arrow), splenomegaly (hash), perigastric varices (asterisk) and esophageal varices (white arrow).

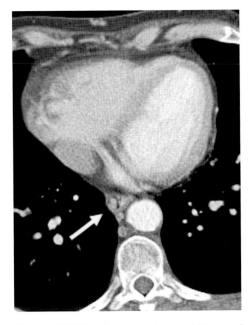

Figure 40.2 Portal venous phase axial image from CT chest and abdomen with intravenous contrast material in a female with alcoholic cirrhosis. Enhancing, tortuous, tubular masses indicative of esophageal varices (white arrow) are smaller than those demonstrated in Figure 40.1.

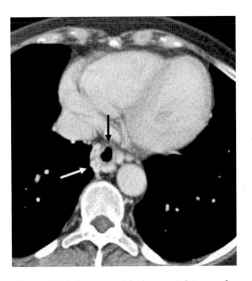

Figure 40.3 Late arterial phase axial image from CT chest and abdomen with intravenous contrast material in a female with primary biliary cirrhosis. The esophageal wall (black arrow) is not thickened nor is the mucosal surface lobulated; therefore, the varices (white arrow) are paraesophageal rather than esophageal (intramural).

Esophageal mural thickening

John Barlow

Imaging description

Esophageal mural thickening is a nonspecific finding by CT chest. Mural thickening may be diffuse, segmental, or focal. It may occur in any segment of the esophagus, although it is more common distally. Intravenous contrast material administration is helpful in the CT evaluation of esophageal mural thickening. Esophagitis is more likely than esophageal carcinoma when uniform, circumferential mural thickening involves a long segment of the esophagus (Figure 41.1) [1]. Esophageal carcinoma is more likely when irregular, asymmetric mural thickening involves a short segment of the esophagus (Figure 41.2). Lymphadenopathy supports the diagnosis of esophageal cancer. Cancers of the mid and upper esophagus typically metastasize to paratracheal lymph nodes; cancers of the lower esophagus typically spread to gastrohepatic ligament lymph nodes [2].

Importance

Esophageal mural thickening is never a normal finding. Since mural thickening is not easily diagnosed by esophagram or by endoscopy, it is important that it be included in the CT chest report. Accurate description of the esophageal mural thickening will encourage referring physicians to consider infection, inflammation, and neoplasm – rather than fibrotic stricture or abnormal motility – as the cause of any dysphagia reported by the patient. Over the last decade, eosinophilic esophagitis has gained greater recognition as a cause of esophagitis (Figure 41.3) [3].

Typical clinical scenario

Dysphagia is a sensitive but nonspecific symptom of pharyngeal or esophageal disease. Esophageal dysphagia usually results from abnormal motility, scarring, esophagitis, or neoplasm; the latter two etiologies cause esophageal mural thickening. Esophagitis commonly results from infection, inflammation, gastroesophageal reflux, caustic ingestion, or radiation. Squamous cell carcinomas of the mid and upper esophagus often occur in individuals with a long history of smoking and alcohol consumption; adenocarcinomas of the distal esophagus often occur in individuals with chronic reflux esophagitis and epithelial metaplasia (Barrett esophagus). Most cases of esophagitis are managed medically; antireflux surgery is available for cases of chronic reflux esophagitis refractory to medical therapy [4]. Esophagectomy remains the mainstay of therapy for both types of esophageal cancer.

Differential diagnosis

Esophageal mural thickening usually results from an infectious, inflammatory, or neoplastic cause: examples from these broad categories are *Candida* esophagitis, reflux esophagitis, eosinophilic esophagitis, squamous cell carcinoma, and adenocarcinoma. Esophageal varices can also cause distal esophageal mural thickening (Figure 41.4). Esophagram and endoscopy often help distinguish between the various etiologies of esophageal mural thickening. For example, both studies can identify the long strictures and luminal rings of eosinophilic esophagitis [5], the plaques of *Candida* esophagitis, and the mucosal ulceration of primary esophageal neoplasm.

Teaching point

Esophageal mural thickening is never a normal finding. Esophagram or endoscopy is usually necessary to sort through the lengthy differential diagnosis for esophageal mural thickening that includes esophageal carcinoma.

REFERENCES

1. Berkovich GY, Levine MS, Miller WT Jr. CT findings in patients with esophagitis. *AJR Am J Roentgenol* 2000; **175**: 1431–1434.

2. Sharma A, Fidias P, Hayman A, et al. Patterns of lymphadenopathy in thoracic malignancies. *Radiographics* 2004; **24**: 419–434.

3. Moawad FJ, Veerappan GR, Wong RK. Eosinophilic esophagitis. *Dig Dis Sci* 2009; **54**: 1818–1828.

4 Kahrilas PJ. Gastroesophageal reflux disease. *JAMA* 1996; **276**: 983–988.

5. Zimmerman SL, Levine MS, Rubesin SE, et al. Idiopathic eosinophilic esophagitis in adults: the ringed esophagus. *Radiology* 2005; **236**: 159–165.

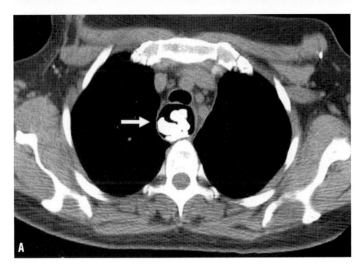

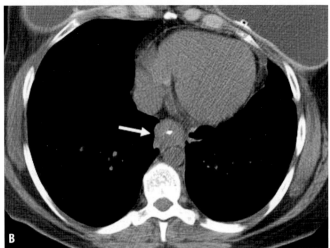

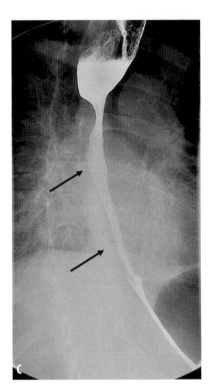

Figure 41.1 A. Axial image from CT chest without intravenous contrast material in a female complaining of dysphagia for 1.5 years. The proximal esophagus is distended and contains globules of barium paste (arrow). B. More inferiorly, circumferential, uniform mural thickening of the distal esophagus surrounds a tiny amount of barium paste in the esophageal lumen (arrow). C. Upright left posterior oblique view from double-contrast esophagram demonstrates the length and severity of this esophageal stricture (arrows). Chronic esophagitis was diagnosed by biopsy. However, an etiology for this inflammation could not be determined.

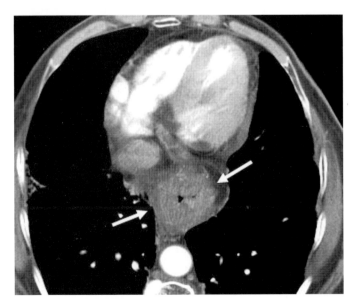

Figure 41.2 Axial image from CT chest with intravenous contrast material, performed for staging purposes, in a female with esophageal cancer demonstrates severe esophageal mural thickening (arrows) that is mildly asymmetric. The mucosal and serosal margins are irregular, the serosal interface with surrounding fat is indistinct, and the thickened esophageal wall enhances heterogeneously.

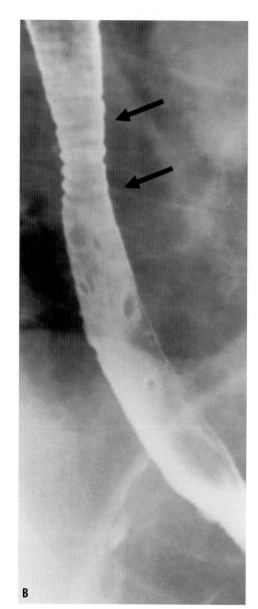

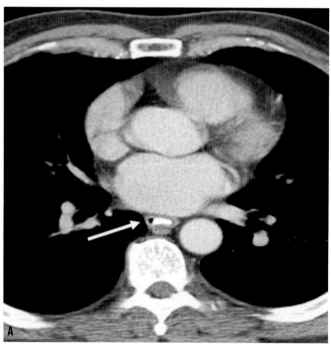

Figure 41.3 A. Axial image from CT neck and chest with intravenous and oral contrast material in a male with solid food dysphagia and a left pulmonary nodule. The wall of the esophagus is mildly thick (arrow), which is a nonspecific finding. **B.** Upright left posterior oblique air-contrast view of the distal esophagus shows that the CT findings result from decreased esophageal caliber and multiple ring-like strictures that give the esophagus a corrugated appearance (arrows). Biopsy of this abnormal region of the esophagus confirmed eosinophilic esophagitis.

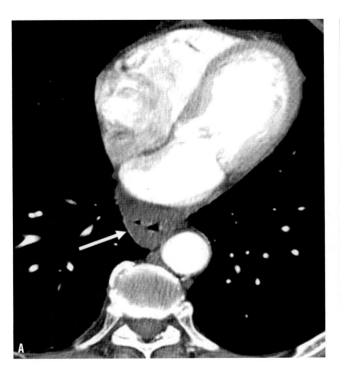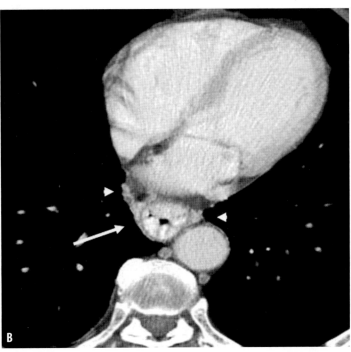

Figure 41.4 A. Axial image of the lower chest from the arterial phase of CT abdomen and pelvis with intravenous contrast material (biphasic imaging). The wall of the distal esophagus is thickened and demonstrates homogeneous low attenuation (arrow). The mucosal surface is lobulated. **B.** Axial image of the lower chest from the portal venous phase of same scan reveals that mural thickening results from numerous, large submucosal enhancing masses (arrow). Longitudinal extension of these masses and the presence of cirrhosis with portal venous hypertension confirmed that they are large esophageal varices. Small paraesophageal varices are also noted (arrowheads).

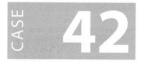

Esophageal dilatation

John Barlow

Imaging description

Nonspecific esophageal distention is the predominant CT finding of achalasia and esophageal scleroderma. Fluoroscopic esophagram demonstrates the key findings of achalasia: absent peristalsis in the lower two-thirds of the esophagus, tapered (beak-like) narrowing of the distal esophagus, and intermittent drainage of barium through the gastroesophageal junction in the upright position (Figure 42.1). Esophageal peristalsis is also absent in patients with scleroderma; however, the esophagram typically demonstrates a distal esophageal stricture (Figure 42.2), secondary to chronic reflux esophagitis, rather than tapered narrowing of the distal esophagus. When present on CT, the pulmonary findings of scleroderma suggest the cause of esophageal dilatation (Figure 42.3).

Importance

Smooth muscle denervation is probably the cause of achalasia [1]; smooth muscle atrophy is likely the cause of scleroderma [2]. Achalasia and esophageal scleroderma are both associated with absent peristalsis in the distal two-thirds of the esophagus. However, the resting pressure of the lower esophageal sphincter (LES) is abnormally high in achalasia and abnormally low in scleroderma. In achalasia the esophagus distends because of functional stenosis of the LES; in scleroderma the esophagus distends because a functionally patulous LES allows chronic gastroesophageal reflux leading to chronic distal esophagitis and eventual fixed, peptic stricture. Pseudoachalasia results from distal esophageal neural plexus dysfunction secondary to invasion by carcinoma or paraneoplastic syndrome [3].

Typical clinical scenario

Achalasia and esophageal scleroderma both cause dysphagia. They also cause stasis of esophageal contents that may result in regurgitation, aspiration pneumonia, pill esophagitis, and *Candida* esophagitis. The risk of squamous cell carcinoma in the achalasia population is about 15 times greater than the risk in the general population [4]. The most significant complication of scleroderma results from the sequence of chronic reflux esophagitis, Barrett esophagus, and adenocarcinoma. Treatment of achalasia by botulinum toxin injection is less successful than treatment by esophageal balloon

dilatation; laparoscopic myotomy with fundoplication is the surgical procedure of choice for achalasia [5].

Differential diagnosis

A distended esophagus by CT may be caused by achalasia, scleroderma, esophageal adenocarcinoma, and distal esophageal stricture of various causes. The differential diagnosis may be narrowed by the presence of interstitial lung disease, favoring scleroderma, or by a distal esophageal mass, favoring esophageal carcinoma. When pulmonary findings of scleroderma are absent, achalasia and scleroderma can be differentiated by esophagram. Achalasia causes tapered narrowing and functional obstruction of the distal esophagus; scleroderma is associated with chronic gastroesophageal reflux that results in focal stricture (mechanical obstruction) of the distal esophagus. Generic chronic reflux esophagitis remains the most common cause of distal esophageal obstruction and esophageal dilatation.

> ## Teaching point
>
> Distention of the esophagus by CT is nonspecific. Further evaluation is usually required before a diagnosis is confirmed. This evaluation requires assessment of esophageal motility and any functional or mechanical obstruction of the distal esophagus. Fluoroscopic esophagram still contributes significantly to this evaluation.

REFERENCES

1. Adler D, Romero Y. Primary esophageal motility disorders. *Mayo Clin Proc* 2001; **76**: 195–200.
2. Roberts CGP, Hummers LK, Ravich WJ, et al. A case-control study of the pathology of esophageal disease in systemic sclerosis (scleroderma). *Gut* 2006; **55**: 1697–1703.
3. Spechler SJ, Castell DO. Classification of esophageal motility abnormalities. *Gut* 2001; **49**: 145–151.
4. Streitz JM, Ellis FH, Gibb SP, et al. Achalasia and squamous cell carcinoma of the esophagus: analysis of 241 patients. *Ann Thorac Surg* 1995; **59**: 1604–1609.
5. Campos G, Vittinghoff E, Rabl C, et al. Endoscopic and surgical treatments for achalasia: a systematic review and meta-analysis. *Ann Surg* 2009; **249**(1): 45–57.

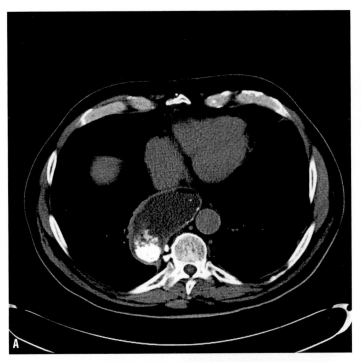

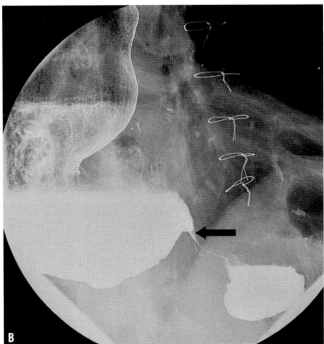

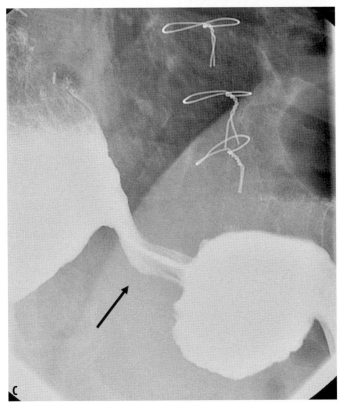

Figure 42.1 A. Axial CT chest without intravenous contrast material in a male complaining of dysphagia. Severely distended esophagus contains air, fluid, and barium. The esophagus is beginning to assume a sigmoid shape that prevents complete emptying even in the upright position. **B.** Upright spot image from double-contrast esophagram demonstrates a distended esophagus and severe, tapered narrowing of the distal esophagus (arrow). Fluoroscopy confirmed the absence of peristalsis in the lower two-thirds of the esophagus. **C.** Upright spot image from double-contrast esophagram demonstrates decreased narrowing of the distal esophagus (arrow) secondary to brief relaxation of the lower esophageal sphincter.

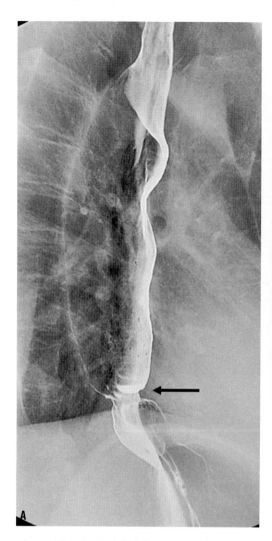
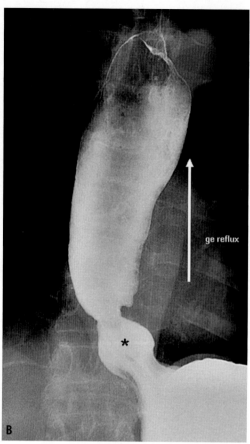

Figure 42.2 A. Upright left posterior oblique double-contrast view of the esophagus in a female complaining of pyrosis, gastroesophageal reflux, regurgitation, and dysphagia. The distal two-thirds of the esophagus are moderately distended. A focal stricture at the gastroesophageal junction (arrow) is located above a small hiatal hernia. **B.** Supine single-contrast view demonstrates gastroesophageal reflux (indicated by long white arrow) and confirms distal esophageal focal stricture. Small sliding hiatal hernia (asterisk) is well demonstrated. No peristalsis was demonstrated in the distal two-thirds of the esophagus when patient drank barium in prone position. These findings are typical of scleroderma complicated by distal esophageal peptic stricture.

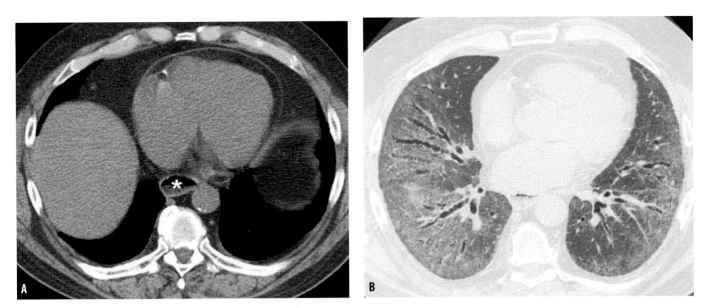

Figure 42.3 A. Axial image from CT chest without intravenous contrast material in a male complaining of dysphagia and dry cough. A mildly to moderately distended distal esophagus contains debris (asterisk). Esophagram did not demonstrate a distal esophageal stricture. **B.** Axial image with lung window settings reveals ground-glass opacities, interstitial fibrosis, and traction bronchiectasis of nonspecific interstitial pneumonitis (NSIP); therefore, the esophageal findings likely result from scleroderma.

Penetrating atheromatous ulcer

Patrick Eiken

Imaging description

Penetrating atheromatous ulcer occurs when ulceration of an atherosclerotic plaque extends through the internal elastic lamina of the aortic wall. On CT, there is ulceration of the aortic wall that extends beyond the expected level of the intima with an overlying bulge in the outer aortic contour (Figures 43.1–43.3). There is usually extensive atherosclerotic disease at and adjacent to the site of ulceration. The arch and descending aorta are the most frequently affected sites. Penetrating ulcer can be categorized according to the Stanford classification for aortic dissection; type A lesions involve the ascending aorta, and type B lesions involve only the descending aorta. Acute expansion of a penetrating ulcer can lead to intramural hematoma. Penetrating ulcer, dissection, and intramural hematoma comprise the "acute aortic syndromes" [1–4].

Importance

The natural history of penetrating aortic ulcer is not entirely clear. Some progress to intramural hematoma, classic dissection, or rupture, while others are asymptomatic and stable. Progression to saccular pseudoaneurysm is common [5, 6]. Asymptomatic patients are generally managed conservatively, while involvement of the ascending aorta or hemodynamic instability are indications for surgical or endovascular intervention [4].

Typical clinical scenario

The entities that cause acute aortic syndrome are clinically indistinguishable from one another. The classic presentation is tearing chest pain radiating to the back in the setting of systemic hypertension. Atypical presentations are common, however, and aortic pathology cannot be reliably excluded by clinical criteria [1]. Imaging evaluation is critical.

Differential diagnosis

Distinguishing penetrating atheromatous ulcer from a simple atheromatous ulceration can be challenging. Features that favor penetrating ulcer include clear extension across a line of intimal calcifications or a focal bulge in the outer aortic contour. Ductus diverticulum creates an aortic outpouching, but has smooth, obtuse borders with the arch and a predictable location. Chronically, pseudoaneurysm from penetrating ulcer may be indistinguishable from pseudoaneurysm secondary to trauma. The presence of extensive atherosclerosis may suggest penetrating ulcer as the culprit.

> ## Teaching point
>
> Penetrating atheromatous ulcer is an increasingly recognized entity in the era of multi-row CT. Penetrating ulcers require imaging follow-up to monitor for progression to intramural hematoma, dissection, pseudoaneurysm, or rupture.

REFERENCES

1. Hayter RG, Rhea JT, Small A, et al. Suspected aortic dissection and other aortic disorders: multi-detector row CT in 373 cases in the emergency setting. *Radiology* 2006; **238**(3): 841–852.
2. Manghat NE, Morgan-Hughes GJ, Roobottom CA. Multi-detector row computed tomography: imaging in acute aortic syndrome. *Clin Radiol* 2005; **60**: 1256–1267.
3. Salvolini L, Renda P, Fiore D, et al. Acute aortic syndromes: role of multi-detector row CT. *Eur J Radiol* 2005; **65**: 350–358.
4. Sundt TM. Intramural hematoma and penetrating atherosclerotic ulcer of the aorta. *Ann Thorac Surg* 2007; **83**: S835–S841.
5. Cho KR, Stanson AW, Potter DD, et al. Penetrating atherosclerotic ulcer of the descending thoracic aorta and arch. *J Thorac Cardiovasc Surg* 2004; **127**: 1393–1401.
6. Tittle SL, Lynch RJ, Cole PE, et al. Midterm follow-up of penetrating ulcer and intramural hematoma of the aorta. *J Thorac Cardiovasc Surg* 2002; **123**: 1051–1059.

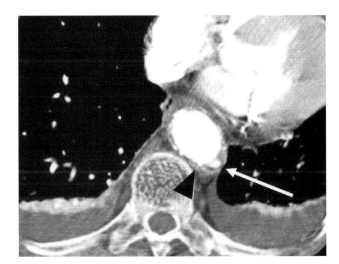

Figure 43.1 Small penetrating ulcer (arrow) extends beyond the intimal calcifications (arrowhead). Note the small bulge in the aortic contour.

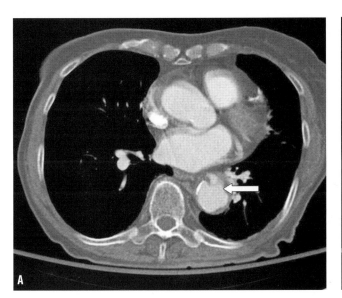
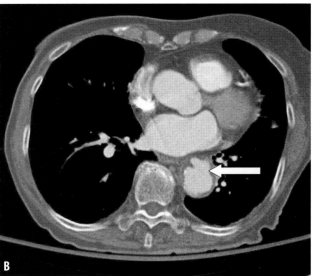

Figure 43.2 A. and **B.** CT images demonstrating a larger penetrating ulcer (arrows). Note extension beyond the expected course of the intimal calcifications and the irregular aortic contour.

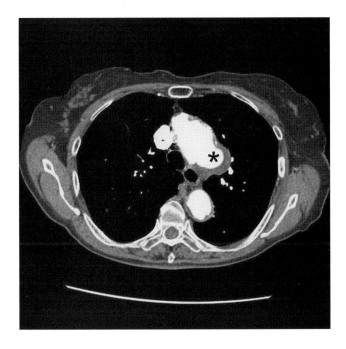

Figure 43.3 Chronic penetrating ulcer has resulted in a large saccular pseudoaneurysm (asterisk) just distal to the left subclavian artery.

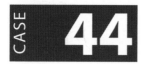

Intramural hematoma

Patrick Eiken

Imaging description

Intramural hematoma (IMH) is characterized by hemorrhage into the media of the aortic wall. It may be spontaneous or secondary to penetrating atheromatous ulcer or trauma. In the absence of trauma, it is included, along with penetrating atheromatous ulcer and dissection, under the clinical term "acute aortic syndrome." IMH is most easily identified on noncontrast CT (Figure 44.1). The typical finding of high-attenuation crescentic or circumferential wall thickening may be masked by contrast material. By definition, communication between the hematoma and the true aortic lumen is absent. The Stanford classification for aortic dissection may also be applied to IMHs: Stanford A IMHs involve the ascending aorta while Stanford B involve only the descending aorta [1–5].

Importance

IMH has an unpredictable clinical course. IMH may resolve without sequelae, but may also progress to aortic dissection, develop ulcer-like projections (Figure 44.2), or rupture [1, 6].

Typical clinical scenario

The entities that cause acute aortic syndrome are clinically indistinguishable from one another. The classic presentation is tearing chest pain radiating to the back in the setting of systemic hypertension. Atypical presentations are common, however, and aortic pathology cannot be reliably excluded by clinical criteria [2]. Imaging evaluation is critical.

Differential diagnosis

Aortic dissection, penetrating atheromatous ulcer, and IMH are related and may coexist in the same patient or evolve one into another. For instance, a penetrating ulcer may cause IMH that subsequently evolves to classic aortic dissection.

Specifically, it can be very difficult to distinguish IMH from an aortic dissection with either a very small entrance flap or a thrombosed lumen. Fortunately, treatment is identical: surgical therapy for type A lesions, and a trial of medical therapy for type B [4]. Other causes of aortic wall thickening, including aortitis, periaortitis, mural thrombus, or atheromatous plaque, may have a similar appearance [4].

Teaching point

IMH is an unpredictable entity that has broad overlap with dissection and penetrating atheromatous ulcer and may also be seen in the setting of blunt trauma. When acute aortic syndrome is suspected, noncontrast images should be obtained prior to CT angiography to avoid masking IMH.

REFERENCES

1. Chao CP, Walker TG, Kalva SP. Natural history and CT appearances of aortic intramural hematoma. *Radiographics* 2009; **29**: 791–804.
2. Hayter RG, Rhea JT, Small A, et al. Suspected aortic dissection and other aortic disorders: multi-detector row CT in 373 cases in the emergency setting. *Radiology* 2006; **238**(3): 841–852.
3. Manghat NE, Morgan-Hughes GJ, Roobottom CA. Multi-detector row computed tomography: imaging in acute aortic syndrome. *Clin Radiol* 2005; **60**: 1256–1267.
4. Salvolini L, Renda P, Fiore D, et al. Acute aortic syndromes: role of multi-detector row CT. *Eur J Radiol* 2008; **65**: 350–358.
5. Sundt TM. Intramural hematoma and penetrating atherosclerotic ulcer of the aorta. *Ann Thorac Surg* 2007; **83**: S835–S841.
6. Bosma MS, Quint LE, Williams DM, et al. Ulcer like projections developing in noncommunicating aortic dissections: CT findings and natural history. *AJR Am J Roentgenol* 2009; **193**(3): 895–905.

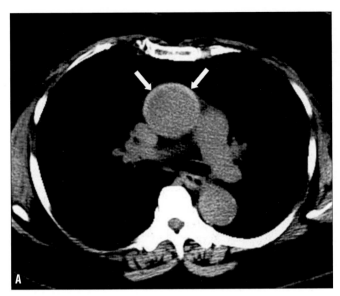 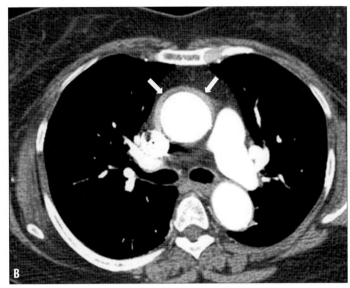

Figure 44.1 A. Noncontrast CT in a 66-year-old woman with chest pain demonstrates high-attenuation wall thickening of the ascending aorta (arrows). **B.** The high-attenuation nature of the aortic wall thickening (arrows) is much more difficult to appreciate following contrast administration.

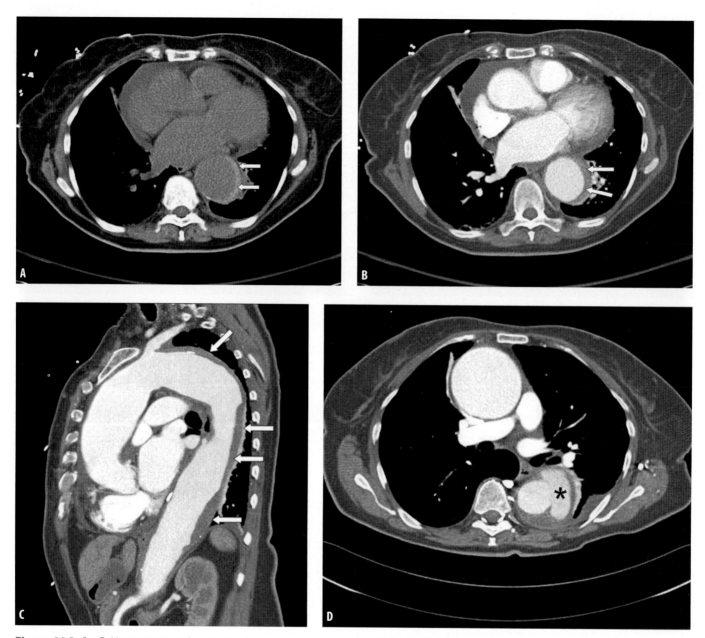

Figure 44.2 A.–C. Noncontrast and contrast-enhanced images in a man with back pain demonstrate typical high-attenuation crescent involving the descending thoracic aorta. **D.** After a one-month trial of medical therapy, follow-up imaging shows enlargement of the aorta with development of a large ulcer-like projection (asterisk).

Aortic dissection

Patrick Eiken

Imaging description

Aortic dissection results from a tear in the aortic intima. Blood flow through the intimal defect results in a true and a false aortic lumen separated by an intimomedial flap. While there is considerable variability, the true lumen is generally smaller than the false lumen and opacifies more quickly following contrast administration (Figure 45.1). With current CT technology, continuity can usually be demonstrated between the true lumen and an unaffected segment of the aorta. The most widely used classification system is the Stanford classification: Stanford A dissection involves the ascending aorta (Figure 45.2) while Stanford B involves only the descending aorta (Figure 45.3). "Acute aortic syndrome" is a term encompassing several related aortic diseases: aortic dissection, intramural hematoma, and penetrating atheromatous ulcer, which have similar clinical features [1–3].

Importance

Stanford A dissection may result in pericardial tamponade or occlusion of coronary, carotid, or vertebral arteries and is usually treated surgically. Type B dissections are generally treated medically, unless there are signs of significant end-organ compromise, such as acute renal failure or bowel ischemia. Either type of dissection may progress to pseudoaneurysm formation or aortic rupture.

Typical clinical scenario

The entities that cause acute aortic syndrome are clinically indistinguishable. The classic presentation is tearing chest pain radiating to the back in the setting of systemic hypertension. Atypical presentations are common, however, and aortic pathology cannot be reliably excluded by clinical criteria [1]. Imaging evaluation is critical.

Differential diagnosis

Identification of an intimomedial flap is pathognomonic for dissection. Distinguishing a dissection with a thrombosed false lumen from intramural hematoma may be impossible. A short-segment dissection and penetrating atheromatous ulcer may be difficult to distinguish from one another. Fortunately, the classification and treatment of the three entities is identical.

Teaching point

Aortic dissection is a potentially deadly cause of acute chest pain. CT is critical in making the diagnosis and determining the appropriate therapy.

REFERENCES

1. Hayter RG, Rhea JT, Small A, et al. Suspected aortic dissection and other aortic disorders: multi-detector row CT in 373 cases in the emergency setting. *Radiology* 2006; **238**(3): 841–852.
2. Manghat NE, Morgan-Hughes GJ, Roobottom CA. Multi-detector row computed tomography: imaging in acute aortic syndrome. *Clin Radiol* 2005; **60**: 1256–1267.
3. Salvolini L, Renda P, Fiore D, et al. Acute aortic syndromes: role of multi-detector row CT. *Eur J Radiol* 2008; **65**: 350–358.

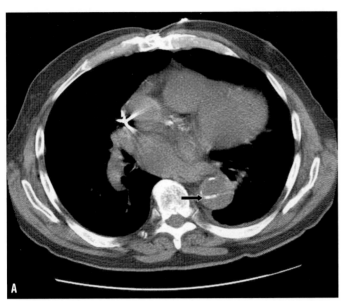
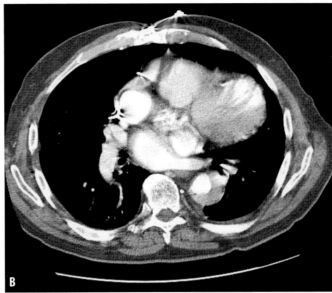

Figure 45.1 **A.** and **B.** Pre- and post-contrast CT images demonstrate dissection of the descending thoracic aorta. True lumen is smaller and more densely contrast opacified, as is typical. Note displaced intimal calcifications (arrow) on the precontrast image **(A)**.

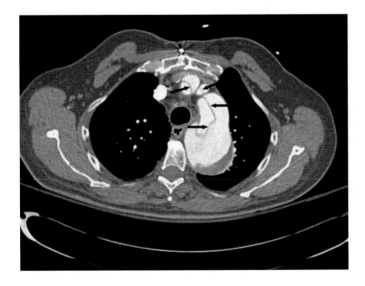

Figure 45.2 Stanford A dissection (arrows) involving the innominate and left common carotid arteries.

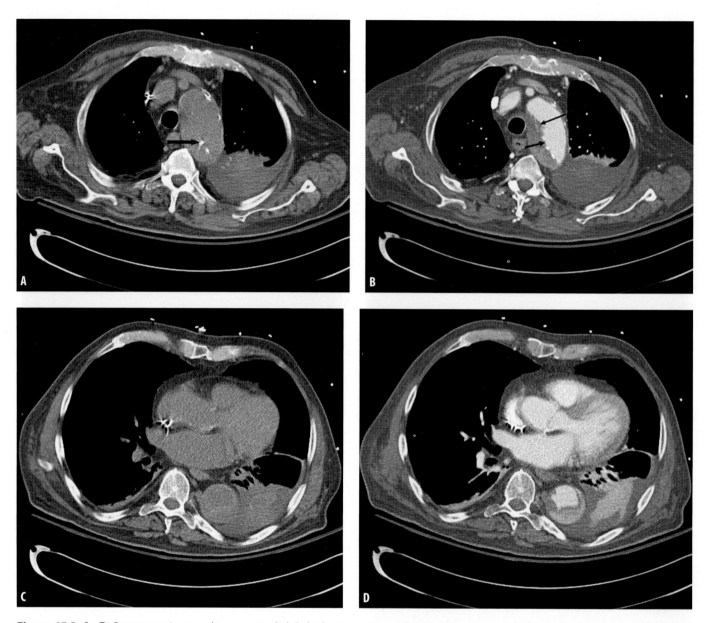

Figure 45.3 A.–D. Precontrast images demonstrate slightly high-attenuation wall thickening suggestive of intramural hematoma **(A, C).** This may represent intramural hematoma progressing to aortic dissection. Note displaced intimal calcification on precontrast image **A** (arrow) and intimal flap on image **B** (arrows). Following contrast, there is opacification of the false lumen distally **(D)** consistent with dissection.

46 Aortic transection

Patrick Eiken

Imaging description

Aortic transection is the most severe form of traumatic aortic injury. In the majority of cases, aortic transection involves all three layers of the aortic wall and results in such rapid exsanguination that the injury is fatal before the patient can present for imaging. Those transections which are seen at imaging consist of contained aortic rupture due to disruption of the intima and media with preservation of the adventitia. Direct CT signs of aortic transection include pseudoaneurysm or contained rupture, abrupt aortic caliber change, irregular aortic contour, or intimal flap (Figures 46.1–46.4). Visualization of frank contrast extravasation is rare. The most common indirect sign is mediastinal hematoma. Aortic injury is most common at the aortic root, the ligamentum arteriosum, and the diaphragm, as the relative fixation of the aorta at these sites creates vulnerability to the shear forces generated in blunt trauma [1, 2].

Importance

Aortic transection is a surgical emergency. Incorrect or delayed diagnosis places the patient at substantial risk of progression to frank aortic rupture and exsanguination. Endovascular repair of aortic transection compares favorably with open repair (Figure 46.4) [3]. To assist in determining the feasibility of endovascular repair it is important to note: the caliber of the aorta proximal and distal to the injury, the length of the injured segment, the type of injury (pseudo-aneurysm, intimal flap), and the presence of any anatomic variants [1]. Proximity to or involvement of arch vessels should also be noted [2, 3].

Typical clinical scenario

Eighty % to 90% of traumatic aortic injuries are the result of motor vehicle collisions.

Differential diagnosis

When direct signs of transection are present, the diagnosis is not in doubt and no further imaging is required. Motion artifact due to breathing or cardiac pulsatility may mimic intimal or contour abnormalities. In these cases, repeat scanning with cardiac gating or conventional angiography may be required.

Teaching point

Aortic transection is an unstable injury that requires rapid identification and definitive surgical or endovascular management.

REFERENCES

1. Mirvis SE, Shanmuganathan K. Diagnosis of blunt traumatic aortic injury 2007: still a nemesis. *Eur J Radiol* 2007; **64**(1): 27–40.
2. Steenburg SD, Ravenel JG, Ikonomidis JS, et al. Acute traumatic aortic injury: imaging evaluation and management. *Radiology* 2008; **248**(3): 748–762.
3. Hoffer EK, Forauer AR, Silas AM, Gemery JM. Endovascular stent-graft or open surgical repair for blunt thoracic aortic trauma: systematic review. *J Vasc Interv Radiol* 2008; **19**: 1153–1164.

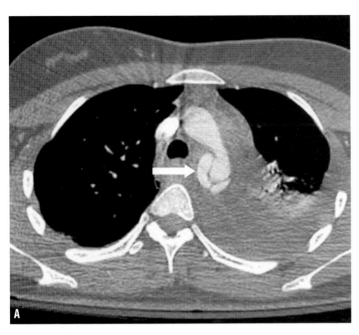
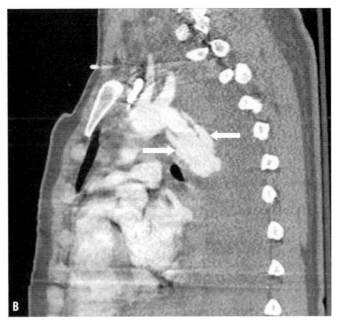

Figure 46.1 A. Axial contrast-enhanced CT image in a woman involved in a motor vehicle collision demonstrates a large pseudoaneurysm (arrow) involving the proximal descending aorta with a large amount of hemorrhage in the mediastinum and left pleural space. **B.** Sagittal reformatted image better demonstrates the longitudinal extent of the injury (arrows).

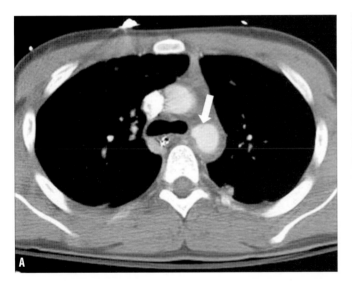
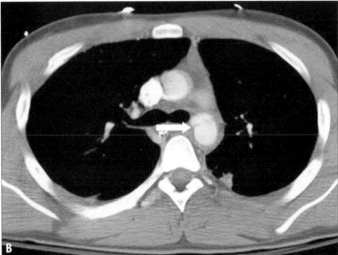

Figure 46.2 A. and **B.** Axial contrast-enhanced CT images in a man involved in a motor vehicle collision demonstrates a small pseudoaneurysm involving the medial aspect of the descending aorta. An intimal flap (arrow) is visible. Note the hematoma surrounding and abutting the aorta. No reformatted images were obtained in this case.

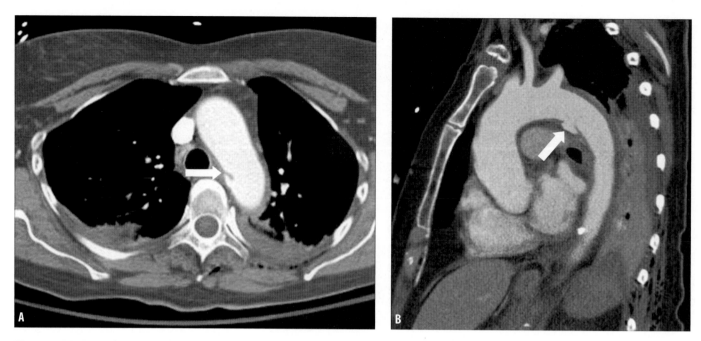

Figure 46.3 A. Axial contrast-enhanced CT image in a man involved in a motor vehicle collision demonstrates a small intimal flap (arrow) and slight contour abnormality of the descending aorta. **B.** Oblique sagittal reformatted image mimics the appearance of conventional angiographic images and more clearly demonstrates the small pseudoaneurysm (arrow).

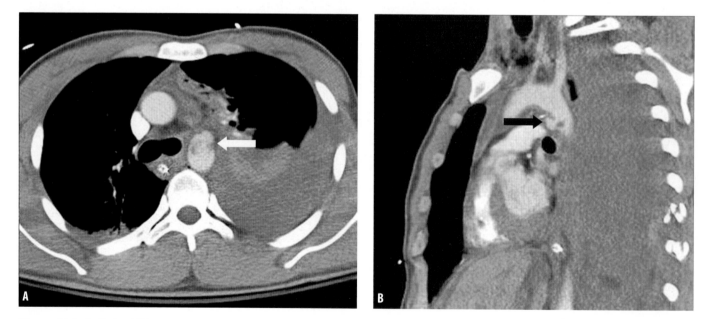

Figure 46.4 A.–F. Axial **(A)** images and sagittal **(B)** and three-dimensional **(C)** reformatted images in a man involved in a motor vehicle collision demonstrate a small pseudoaneurysm (arrow). Conventional angiographic images were obtained during endovascular repair before **(D)** and after **(E)** stent graft deployment. Follow-up CT **(F)** demonstrates the stent graft in place and exclusion of the pseudoaneurysm.

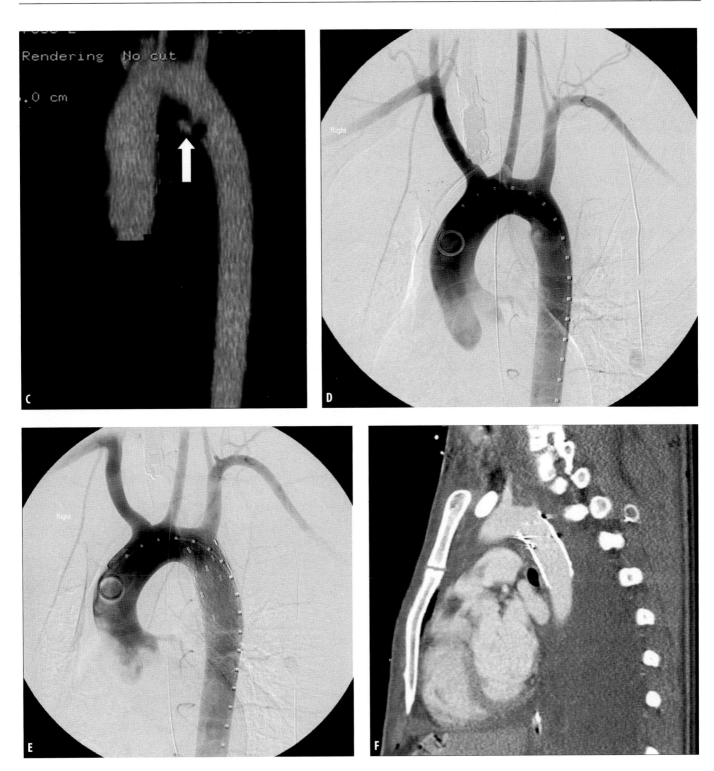

Figure 46.4 (cont.)

47 Coarctation and pseudocoarctation of the aorta

Patrick Eiken

Imaging description

Coarctation of the aorta is a congenital defect thought to result from incorporation of tissue from the ductus arteriosus into the wall of the aorta. Regression of the ductal tissue results in focal narrowing and kinking of the proximal descending aorta [1, 2]. If the obstruction is severe enough, blood flow to the lower body may become dependent on collateral flow, usually via the intercostal or internal mammary arteries (Figure 47.1). Dilatation of the intercostal arteries can result in erosion of the inferior aspect of the ribs and the classic chest radiographic finding of rib notching [3]. Pseudocoarctation refers to mild cases of narrowing without significant collateral flow (Figure 47.2). The pressure gradient across the narrowed segment in pseudocoarctation is <25 mmHg by definition [4].

Importance

Coarctation of the aorta is seen in association with a number of syndromes and intracardiac congenital defects. In adults, coarctation can be associated with aortic or intercostal aneurysm formation, aortic dissection, and intracranial berry aneurysm formation [2].

Typical clinical scenario

The classic clinical scenario in adults is hypertension when the blood pressure is measured in the upper extremities, but diminished or absent pulses in the lower extremities. Coarctation of the aorta may also come to clinical attention due to murmur or claudication. Treatment is by surgical bypass or endovascular dilatation of the stenotic segment.

Differential diagnosis

The appearance is quite characteristic, particularly in the presence of prominent collateral vessels. Marked aortic tortuosity in an elderly, kyphotic patient may mimic the kinked appearance.

> ### Teaching point
>
> Coarctation of the aorta is a common congenital obstructive lesion of the aorta. Its sequelae are related to either hypertension or associated lesions. MRI and CT are useful in evaluating the degree of collateral flow and defining the anatomy prior to surgical or endovascular repair.

REFERENCES

1. Knauth Meadows A, Ordovas K, Higgins CB, Reddy GP. Magnetic resonance imaging in the adult with congenital heart disease. *Semin Roentgenol* 2008; **43**(3): 246–258.
2. Markle BM, Cross RR. Cross-sectional imaging in congenital anomalies of the heart and great vessels: magnetic resonance imaging and computed tomography. *Semin Roentgenol* 2004; **39**(2): 234–262.
3. Jaffe RB. Radiographic manifestations of congenital anomalies of the aortic arch. *Radiol Clin North Am* 1991; **29**(2): 319–334.
4. Wang WB, Lin GM. Pseudocoarctation and coarctation. *Int J Cardiol* 2009; **133**(2): e62–e64.

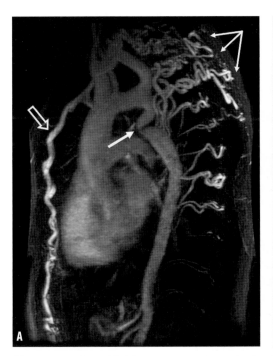
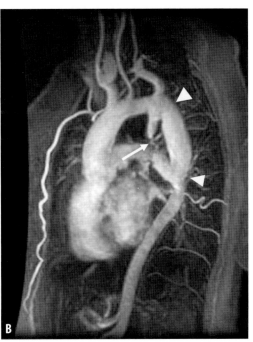

Figure 47.1 A. and **B.** Maximum intensity projection (MIP) images from gadolinium-enhanced MRAs before **(A)** and after **(B)** aortic coarctation (arrow) repair. Pre-repair image demonstrates marked enlargement of the internal mammary arteries (open arrow) and intercostal arteries (trifurcated arrow). These vessels are less prominent following repair. Arrowheads indicate the proximal and distal ends of the surgical graft bridging the site of coarctation.

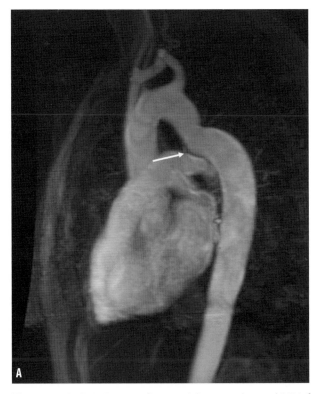
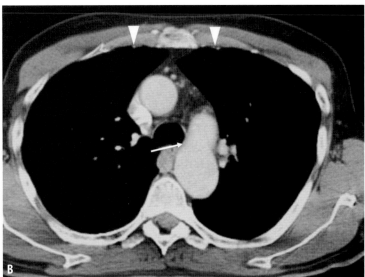

Figure 47.2 A. MIP image from gadolinium-enhanced MRA from a patient with pseudocoarctation demonstrates marked tortuosity and focal narrowing (arrow) of the aorta, but none of the prominent collaterals seen in Figure 47.1A. **B.** Contrast-enhanced CT in the same patient also demonstrates focal narrowing and slight post-stenotic dilatation (arrow). Note the normal caliber internal mammary arteries (arrowheads).

Patrick Eiken

Imaging description

In double aortic arch, the ascending aorta divides into left and right arches (Figure 48.1). Usually, both arches are patent; in a minority of cases, a portion of the smaller arch is atretic. The left arch is generally in a normal position relative to mediastinal structures, passing anterior and to the left of the trachea and esophagus. The right arch usually extends further cephalad than the left arch, and it passes to the right and posterior to the trachea and esophagus. In 70–80% of cases the right arch is larger [1–3]. A subclavian and a common carotid artery arise from each arch. The two arches combine in the upper chest to form the descending aorta, which usually lies in a normal position to the left of the spine [1–4].

Importance

Double aortic arch is the most common complete vascular ring. The two arches encircle the trachea and esophagus, which can result in tracheal or esophageal narrowing. Associated congenital intracardiac defects are rare [1–4].

Typical clinical scenario

Symptoms of dysphagia, stridor, or recurrent respiratory infections generally lead to discovery of this congenital anomaly within the first 6 months of life. If tracheal or esophageal compression is less severe, double aortic arch may be discovered incidentally in adults. Surgical treatment consists of ligation of the smaller of the two arches [1].

Differential diagnosis

The appearance on cross-sectional imaging is diagnostic. After surgical correction, the branching pattern may mimic other aortic anomalies. For example, remote repair with ligation of the left arch may be confused with a right arch with mirror image branching (Figure 48.2).

> ### Teaching point
>
> Double aortic arch, while rare, is the most common complete vascular ring. The radiologist should note any mass effect on the trachea or esophagus and the relative size and position of the two arches to aid in surgical planning.

REFERENCES

1. Baraldi R, Sala S, Bighi S, Mannella P. Vascular ring due to double aortic arch: a rare cause of dysphagia. *Eur J Radiol Extra* 2004; **52**: 21–24.
2. Jaffe RB. Radiographic manifestations of congenital anomalies of the aortic arch. *Radiol Clin North Am* 1991; **29**(2): 319–334.
3. Markle BM, Cross RR. Cross-sectional imaging in congenital anomalies of the heart and great vessels: magnetic resonance imaging and computed tomography. *Semin Roentgenol* 2004; **39**(2): 234–262.
4. Türkvatan A, Büyükbayraktar FG, Ölçer T, Cumhur T. Congenital anomalies of the aortic arch: evaluation with use of multidetector computed tomography. *Korean J Radiol* 2009; **10**: 176–184.

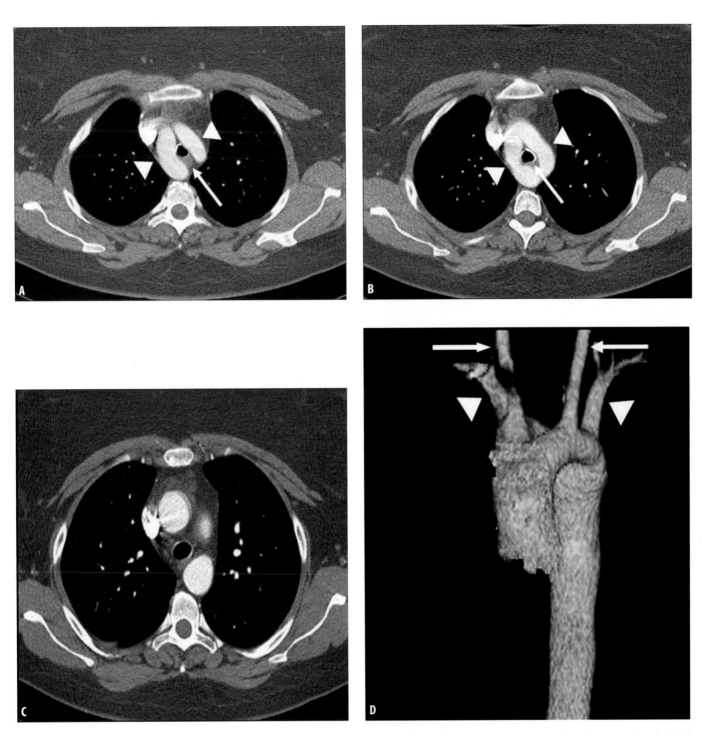

Figure 48.1 A.–D. CT angiogram demonstrates a double aortic arch with approximately equal-sized right and left arches (arrowheads, **A, B**). Trachea is narrowed slightly and esophagus (arrow) is compressed (**A, B**). Ascending aorta and descending aorta caudad to the level of the arches are normal (**C**). Three-dimensional reconstruction (**D**) demonstrates a subclavian artery (arrowhead) and a common carotid artery (arrow) arising from each arch.

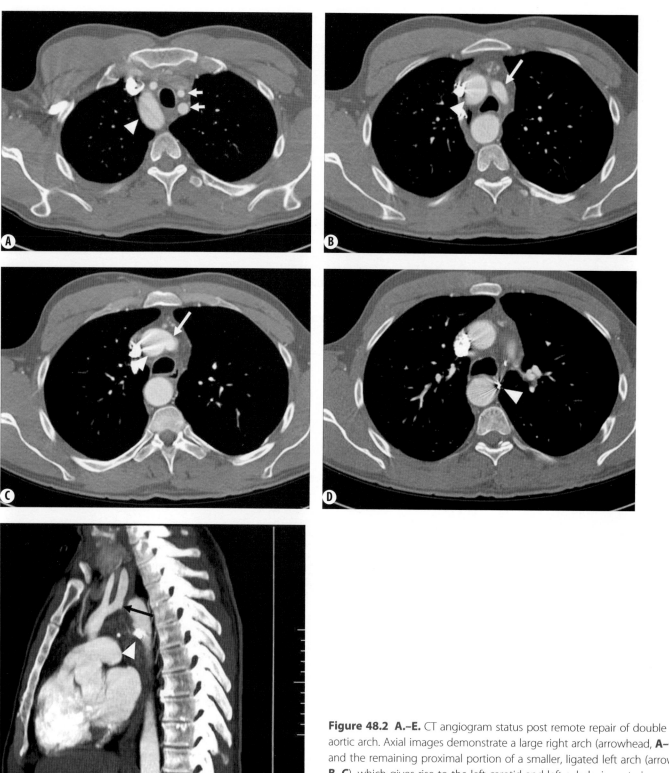

Figure 48.2 A.–E. CT angiogram status post remote repair of double aortic arch. Axial images demonstrate a large right arch (arrowhead, **A–C**) and the remaining proximal portion of a smaller, ligated left arch (arrow, **B, C**), which gives rise to the left carotid and left subclavian arteries (short arrows, **A**). Appearance is now analogous to right arch with mirror image branching. Surgical clips are visible adjacent to the descending aorta at the distal ligation site (arrowhead, **D**). Sagittal maximum intensity projection image (**E**) demonstrates the relationship of the ligated end of the left arch (black arrow) and the surgical clips (arrowhead).

Right aortic arch

Patrick Eiken

Imaging description

In right aortic arch (RAA), the normal, left-sided aortic arch is absent. Instead, the aortic arch lies to the right of the trachea and esophagus. This anomaly has two major variants: RAA with aberrant left subclavian artery and RAA with mirror image branching. In RAA with aberrant left subclavian artery the branching pattern of the arch vessels is left common carotid, right common carotid, and right subclavian artery. The aberrant left subclavian artery arises distally from the proximal descending aorta and passes posterior to the trachea and esophagus (Figures 49.1 and 49.2). In RAA with mirror image branching the branching order is left innominate artery, right common carotid, and right subclavian artery (Figures 49.3 and 49.4) [1–3].

Importance

RAA with aberrant left subclavian artery is the more common variant and has a low association with congenital intracardiac defects. It may rarely form a complete vascular ring with a left ligamentum arteriosus and result in stridor or dysphagia (Figure 49.2). RAA with mirror image branching is often associated with intracardiac defects, commonly tetralogy of Fallot and truncus arteriosus [3].

Typical clinical scenario

RAA with aberrant left subclavian artery is often asymptomatic and discovered incidentally. RAA with mirror image branching is often discovered in infancy, usually due to associated cardiac anomalies.

Differential diagnosis

As demonstrated in Case 48 (Figure 48.2), a surgically repaired double aortic arch may be nearly indistinguishable from a right aortic arch with mirror image branching. Otherwise, the appearance on cross-sectional imaging is diagnostic.

Teaching point

RAA is a relatively common congenital anomaly. The most common variant, RAA with aberrant left subclavian artery can rarely form a complete vascular ring. A less common variant, RAA with mirror image branching, has a very high association with complex congenital heart disease.

REFERENCES

1. Jaffe RB. Radiographic manifestations of congenital anomalies of the aortic arch. *Radiol Clin North Am* 1991; **29**(2): 319–334.
2. Markle BM, Cross RR. Cross-sectional imaging in congenital anomalies of the heart and great vessels: magnetic resonance imaging and computed tomography. *Semin Roentgenol* 2004; **39**(2): 234–262.
3. Türkvatan A, Büyükbayraktar FG, Olçer T, Cumhur T. Congenital anomalies of the aortic arch: evaluation with use of multidetector computed tomography. *Korean J Radiol* 2009; **10**: 176–184.

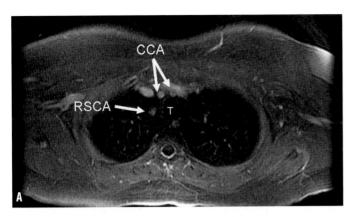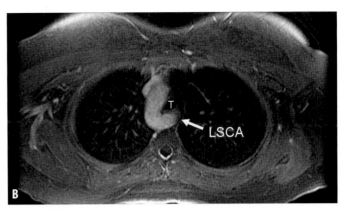

Figure 49.1 A. and **B.** Right arch with aberrant subclavian artery: gadolinium bolus MRA demonstrates both common carotid arteries (CCA) and the right subclavian (RSCA) artery arising from the proximal right arch. Aberrant left subclavian artery (LSCA) arises from the distal arch/proximal descending aorta and passes posterior to the trachea (T) and esophagus.

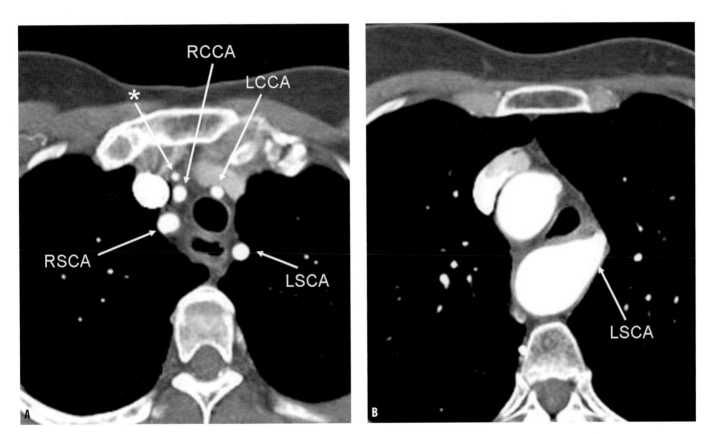

Figure 49.2 A. and **B.** Right arch with aberrant subclavian artery: CT angiogram demonstrates the relationship of the left subclavian (LSCA), left common carotid (LCCA), right common carotid (RCCA), and right subclavian (RSCA) arteries in the superior mediastinum. The asterisk denotes contrast reflux into an inferior thyroid vein. Left subclavian artery arises distally from a dilated diverticulum of Kommerell.

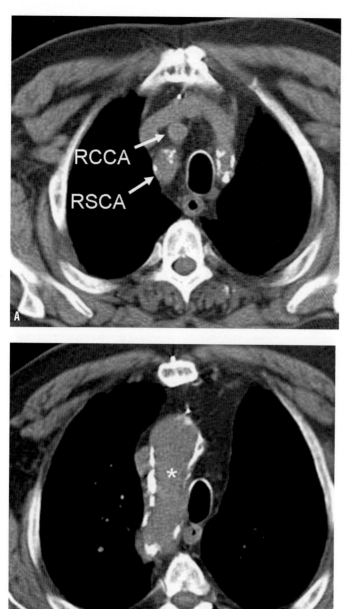

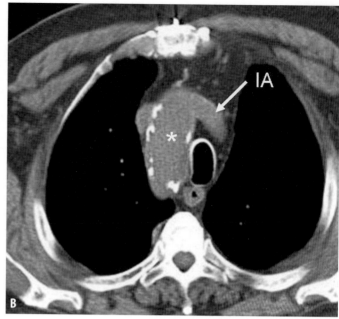

Figure 49.3 A.–C. Right arch with mirror image branching: noncontrast CT demonstrates a left innominate artery (IA). Right common carotid (RCCA) and subclavian (RSCA) arteries arise directly from the right arch (asterisk).

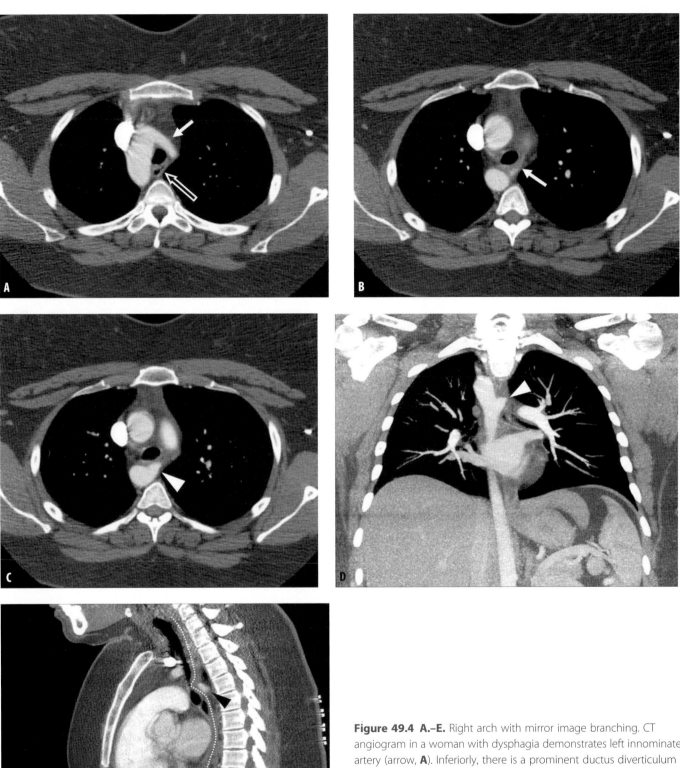

Figure 49.4 A.–E. Right arch with mirror image branching. CT angiogram in a woman with dysphagia demonstrates left innominate artery (arrow, **A**). Inferiorly, there is a prominent ductus diverticulum (arrowhead, **C**) and calcification of much of the ligamentum arteriosum (arrow, **B**). Note that the esophagus (open arrow) is visible on image A, but entirely effaced on **B** and **C.** Coronal and sagittal maximum intensity projection images demonstrate the ductus diverticulum (arrowhead, **D** and **E**) and its mass effect on the esophagus (dotted line, **E**).

Pulmonary sling

Patrick Eiken

Imaging description

In pulmonary sling, the left pulmonary artery arises from the right pulmonary artery. The anomalous left pulmonary artery passes posteriorly, between the trachea and esophagus, to supply the left lung (Figure 50.1) [1–3]. Pulmonary sling is associated with the presence of complete tracheal rings in 50–65% of cases [2]. The complete rings are usually narrowed. This constellation of findings is known as ring-sling complex and can cause life-threatening respiratory complications in infants.

Importance

While rare in asymptomatic adults, pulmonary sling may mimic a mediastinal mass on chest radiograph.

Typical clinical scenario

Typically pulmonary sling is discovered and surgically repaired in infancy due to respiratory compromise from the aberrant vessel or due to the high association with tracheo-bronchial and intracardiac defects.

Differential diagnosis

The cross-sectional imaging appearance is diagnostic. When this anomaly is encountered, the study should be scrutinized for other congenital defects.

Teaching point

A rare anomaly, pulmonary sling may present as a mediastinal mass in adults who are either asymptomatic or have respiratory complaints.

REFERENCES

1. Castañer E, Gallardo X, Rimola J, et al. Congenital and acquired pulmonary artery anomalies in the adult: radiologic overview. *Radiographics* 2006; **26**(2): 349–371.
2. Fiore AC, Brown JW, Weber TR, Turrentine MW. Surgical treatment of pulmonary artery sling and tracheal stenosis. *Ann Thorac Surg* 2005; **79**(1): 38–46.
3. Zylak CJ, Eyler WR, Spizarny DL, Stone CH. Developmental lung anomalies in the adult: radiologic-pathologic correlation. *Radiographics* 2002; **22** Spec No: S25–S43.

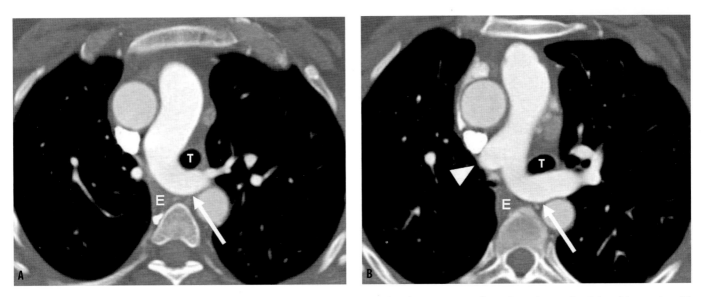

Figure 50.1 A. and **B.** Axial contrast-enhanced CT images demonstrate the left pulmonary artery (arrow) passing to the right of the trachea (T), then between the trachea and esophagus (E). The arrowhead (Figure 50.1B) indicates the origin of the right pulmonary artery.

Takayasu's arteritis

Patrick Eiken

Imaging description

Takayasu's arteritis (TA) is clinically classified as a large-vessel vasculitis, as it largely affects the aorta and its major branches and the pulmonary arteries. TA is a disease of young patients, and is often imaged using MRI to avoid repeated radiation exposure. Typical imaging findings include arterial wall thickening early in the disease (Figure 51.1), followed by stenosis, occlusion, and aneurysmal dilatation in the late phase [1–3]. The most commonly involved vessels are the proximal subclavian and carotid arteries (Figure 51.2) [1]. The pulmonary arteries are affected in approximately 50–80% of cases and may demonstrate mural calcification late in the disease [2]. The lesions of TA are positive on FDG-PET (Figure 51.3), but the utility of PET in monitoring disease activity has yet to be conclusively proven [1].

Importance

Early TA causes nonspecific constitutional symptoms. Recognition of arterial wall thickening may aid early diagnosis. Late in the disease, symptoms are related to vascular occlusion and imaging is useful in evaluating vascular patency and in surgical planning.

Typical clinical scenario

Patients with TA are generally less than 40 years old. The classic presentation is nonspecific constitutional symptoms progressing to signs of vascular occlusion, such as absent pulses or claudication.

Differential diagnosis

Giant cell arteritis may have similar arterial findings, but occurs in patients over 50 years old. Wall thickening secondary to atherosclerosis is usually irregular, unlike the smooth, homogeneous wall thickening associated with vasculitides.

Teaching point

Arterial wall thickening, long-segment stenoses, and occlusions in a young patient suggest Takayasu's arteritis.

REFERENCES

1. Blockmans D, Bley T, Schmidt W. Imaging for large-vessel vasculitis. *Curr Opin Rheumatol* 2009; **21**(1): 19–28.
2. Castañer E, Alguersuari A, Gallardo X, et al. When to suspect pulmonary vasculitis: radiologic and clinical clues. *Radiographics* 2010; **30**(1): 33–53.
3. Khandelwal N, Kalra N, Garg MK, et al. Multidetector CT angiography in Takayasu arteritis. *Eur J Radiol* 2009; **77**(2): 369–374. doi:10.1016/j.ejrad.2009.08.001.

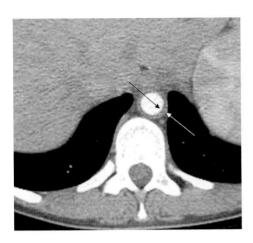

Figure 51.1 Post-contrast CT demonstrates wall thickening of the descending aorta (arrows) in this patient with Takayasu arteritis.

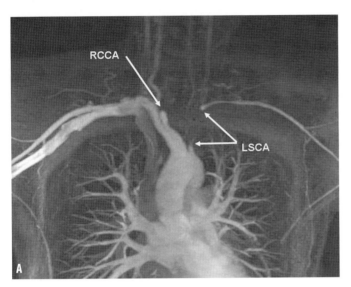

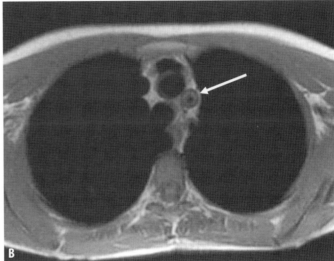

Figure 51.2 A. Maximum intensity projection image from a gadolinium bolus MRA demonstrates long-segment occlusion of the left subclavian artery (LSCA). Both carotid arteries are occluded. The proximal stump of the right common carotid (RCCA) is visible. **B.** Black blood MR sequence in the same patient demonstrates marked wall thickening of the occluded left common carotid (arrow). Mild wall thickening of the innominate artery and LSCA is also visible.

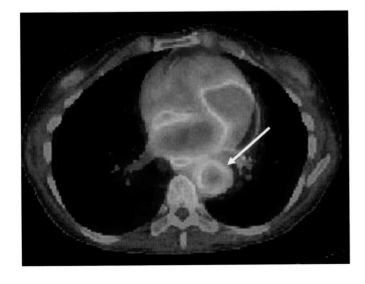

Figure 51.3 Fused image from a PET/CT exam demonstrates moderate hypermetabolism within the wall of the descending thoracic aorta (arrow).

CASE 52

Unilateral absence of a pulmonary artery (UAPA)

Anne-Marie Sykes

Imaging description

Absence or proximal interruption of either the right or left pulmonary artery usually occurs within 1 cm of its origin from the main pulmonary artery [1]. More distal segments of the arteries in the hila are usually present, but are usually diminutive and are supplied by systemic collateral vessels which can arise from bronchial, internal mammary, and intercostal arteries. CT shows the abnormal termination of the pulmonary artery and the collateral vessels supplying the lung (Figure 52.1). Other findings include diminished pulmonary vascularity on that side, decreased size of the affected lung, and a contracted hemithorax. There is also resultant hyperexpansion of the contralateral lung.

Left-sided UAPA is often associated with congential anomalies (Figure 52.2), particularly cardiac anomalies such as tetralogy of Fallot and septal defects. Right-sided UAPA is infrequently associated with other congenital anomalies, and is often referred to as isolated UAPA (IUAPA).

Importance

When associated with congenital anomalies, surgical intervention for those anomalies is usually necessary. UAPA should not be confused with the complex congenital syndrome of pulmonary atresia, in which the pulmonary valve orifice fails to develop.

Typical clinical scenario

Most patients present in the first year of life with dyspnea or recurrent pulmonary infections. Some patients may be asymptomatic, however, and the diagnosis may not be made until adolescence or adulthood when chest radiographs or CT scans are obtained for other indications. This later presentation usually occurs in patients without associated cardiac anomalies (IUAPA). Occasionally hemoptysis can occur, which is due to rupture of hypertrophied vascular collaterals (a result of systemic-to-pulmonary arterial shunting). Approximately 50% experience recurrent pulmonary infections [2]. Pulmonary hypertension occurs in a small number of patients.

Differential diagnosis

In patients with IUAPA, the diagnosis may be difficult on the chest radiograph as other conditions such as Swyer-James-MacLeod syndrome, pulmonary thromboembolic disease, and fibrosing mediastinitis can mimic the appearance of IUAPA. However, the CT findings showing the atretic pulmonary artery segment and the vascular collaterals are typically diagnostic.

Teaching point

Consider IUAPA in a patient who presents with recurrent chest infections or hemoptysis, and chest radiograph findings of contracted hemithorax, decreased unilateral pulmonary vascularity, and hyperexpanded contralateral hemithorax. CT chest is useful in demonstrating the atretic portion and associated vascular collaterals, and can exclude the other differential considerations.

REFERENCES

1. Rubin GD, Rofsky NM. (eds.) *CT and MR Angiography: Comprehensive Vascular Assessment.* Philadelphia, PA: Lippincott Williams & Wilkins, 2009.
2. Yui MWC, Le Dv, Leung Y, Ooi CGC. Radiological features of isolated unilateral absence of the pulmonary artery, a case report. *J HK Coll Radiol* 2001; **4**: 277–280.

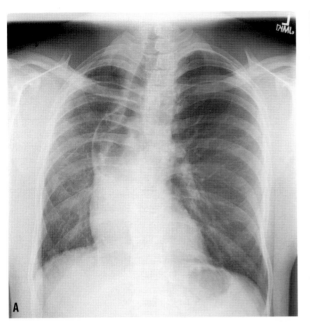

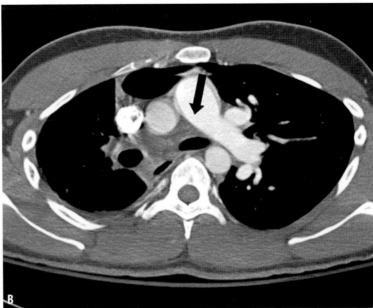

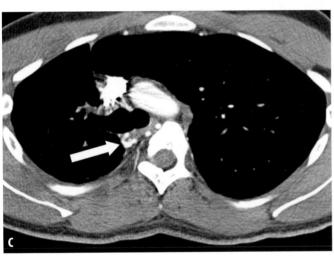

Figure 52.1 **A.** Right-sided unilateral absence of a pulmonary artery (UAPA). Chest radiograph shows asymmetry of the hemithoraces due to small right hemithorax and compensatory hyperexpansion of the left lung. The central left pulmonary arteries are visible, but the right central pulmonary vessels cannot be discerned. **B.** Right-sided UAPA. CT scan of patient in Figure 52.1 shows no right pulmonary artery arising from the main pulmonary artery (arrow). **C.** Right-sided UAPA. Blood supply to the right lung is via hypertrophied bronchial arteries (white arrow).

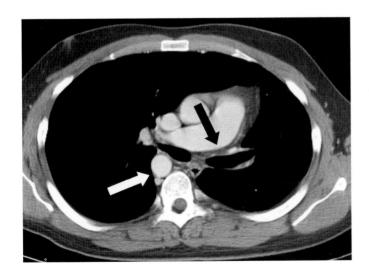

Figure 52.2 Left-sided UAPA. CT scan shows no left pulmonary artery arising from its expected location from the main pulmonary artery (black arrow). Also note the right-sided aorta (white arrow) secondary to a right-sided aortic arch. Left-sided UAPA is more frequently associated with congenital anomalies.

Partial anomalous pulmonary venous return (PAPVR)

Anne-Marie Sykes

Imaging description

In partial anomalous pulmonary venous return (PAPVR) there is an abnormal connection between the draining veins of one or more lobes to a systemic venous structure that drains into the right side of the heart, resulting in a left-to-right shunt. On CT the anomalous venous return is diagnosed based on recognizing the abnormal course of the intraparenchymal pulmonary vein. There are three common patterns of anomalous drainage:

1. Anomalous right superior pulmonary venous drainage to the superior vena cava (SVC) – on CT the right upper lobe drains into the SVC, usually near the SVC/right atrial (RA) junction (Figure 53.1).
2. Anomalous left superior pulmonary venous return to the left brachiocephalic (innominate) vein – on CT a vertical vein is seen coursing lateral to the aortic arch and aortopulmonary window. Blood flow is caudocranial (Figure 53.2).
3. Anomalous right lower lobe drainage into the inferior vena cava (IVC), portal vein, or hepatic vein – on CT the right lower lobe vein courses inferomedially to connect with one of these structures (Figures 53.3 and 53.4).

Importance

All forms of PAPVR result in a left-to right shunt. In addition:

1. Anomalous right superior pulmonary venous drainage to the SVC near the SVC/RA junction is commonly (up to 90%) associated with a sinus venosus defect [1].
2. Anomalous left superior pulmonary venous return to the left brachiocephalic (innominate) vein can sometimes be mistaken for a persistent left SVC; however, with persistent left SVC CT will show two vessels in the left hilar region (the left SVC and left pulmonary vein) whereas only one vessel is seen in this location (small lingual vein) with left

superior PAPVR. In addition, the persistent left SVC usually drains into the coronary sinus [2].
3. Anomalous right lower lobe drainage, when associated with a hypoplastic right lung and right pulmonary artery, mediastinal shift to the right, and systemic arterial supply to the right lung, is known as the Scimitar syndrome.

Typical clinical scenario

As an isolated anomaly in an otherwise healthy individual, partial anomalous return is usually asymptomatic [1], and noted incidentally on CT chest performed for other indications.

Differential diagnosis

The left superior PAPVR should not be mistaken for a persistent left-sided SVC.

> ### Teaching point
>
> Patients with PAPVR are most often asymptomatic, and the anomalous veins are found incidentally on CT performed for other reasons. Knowledge of the draining pattern, associations, and mimics is useful in identifying these anomalous veins.

REFERENCES

1. Rubin, GD, Rofsky NM. (eds.) *CT and MR Angiography: Comprehensive Vascular Assessment.* Philadelphia, PA: Lippincott Williams & Wilkins, 2009.
2. Dillon EH, Camputaro C. Partial anomalous pulmonary venous drainage of the left upper lobe vs. duplication of the superior vena cava: distinction based on CT findings. *AJR Am J Roentgenol* 1993; **160**: 375–379.

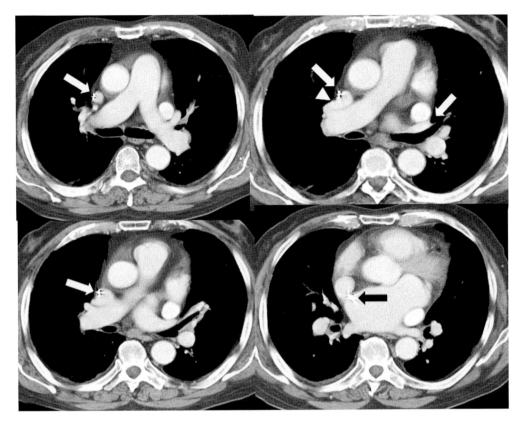

Figure 53.1 Partial anomalous
pulmonary venous return (PAPVR),
with sinus venosus defect. The
arrowhead shows the right
superior pulmonary vein draining
into the SVC near the SVC/RA
junction. Small white arrows show
a pacer wire in the SVC, crossing
over into the left atrium through a
sinus venosus defect (black arrow).
Note also the presence of a
left-sided SVC.

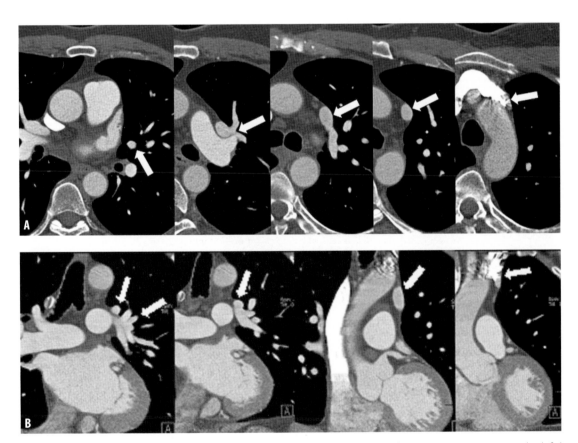

Figure 53.2 A. Partial anomalous pulmonary venous return – left superior pulmonary venous return to the left brachiocephalic vein via a
vertical vein (white arrows). Note the similarity to persistent left SVC. **B.** Partial anomalous pulmonary venous return – left superior pulmonary
venous return to the left brachiocephalic vein via a vertical vein (white arrows). Note the similarity to persistent left SVC.

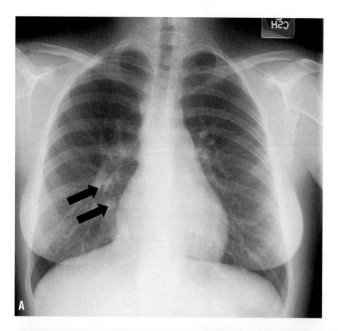

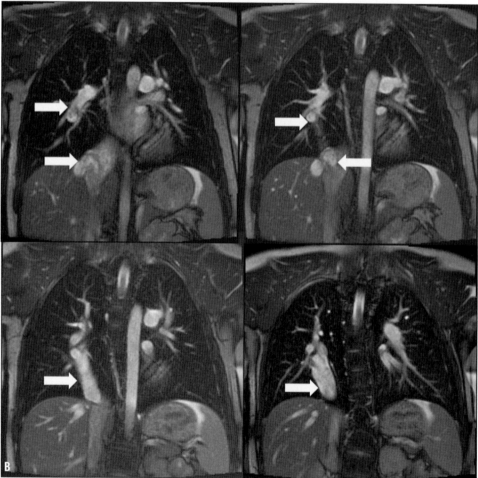

Figure 53.3 A. Partial anomalous pulmonary venous return (PAPVR) Scimitar syndrome. The chest radiograph shows a vertically oriented tubular structure in the right lower chest medially (black arrows). The chest radiograph is somewhat atypical as the right hemithorax is not small. **B.** Partial anomalous pulmonary venous return (PAPVR) Scimitar syndrome. MRI of the chest shows the anomalous right pulmonary vein draining the lung and entering the IVC at the level of the diaphragm (arrows). The IVC and hepatic veins are dilated.

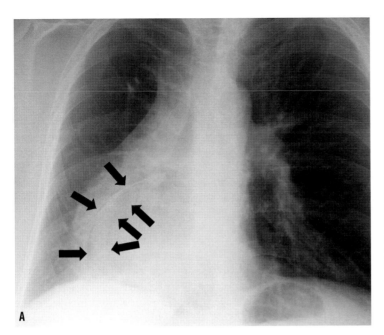
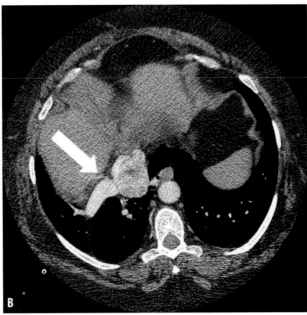

Figure 53.4 A. Scimitar syndrome. Chest radiograph shows small right hemithorax with dextroposition of the heart and a curvilinear tubular structure in the right lower chest (arrows), typical of Scimitar syndrome. **B.** Scimitar syndrome. Enhanced CT shows a large vein in the right lower chest draining into the suprahepatic IVC (white arrow).

Pulmonary arteriovenous malformations (PAVMs)

Anne-Marie Sykes

Imaging description

Arteriovenous malformations (AVMs) are abnormal connections between arteries and veins. Pulmonary AVMs (PAVMs) can be virtually any size, but are most typically between 1 and 5 cm. They can be single or multiple, and can be found anywhere in the lungs, although they are slightly more prevalent in the lower lobes [1]. The AVM consists of one or more feeding arteries and a draining vein, connected by either a large single sac, a plexiform mass of dilated vascular channels, or a direct artery–vein connection which is dilated and often tortuous. The lesions usually appear as nodular opacities on CT and the feeding arteries and draining veins are typically identifiable as tubular structures medial to the nodular opacity (Figures 54.1–54.3). Contrast is usually not needed to make the diagnosis, but when administered PAVMs usually enhance intensely, although this may not be visible in very tiny or thrombosed PAVMs.

Importance

Most patients (70–90%) with pulmonary AVMs have hereditary hemorrhagic telangiectasia (HHT), also known as Osler-Weber-Rendu syndrome. In this syndrome, these lesions are present at birth, however, they usually are not clinically apparent until adulthood. CT is useful in confirming the diagnosis of PAVM by demonstrating the feeding and draining vessels, characterizing the AVMs as simple (single feeding vessel, more straightforward to treat) or complex (multiple feeding vessels), and for measurement of feeding vessel size since embolization therapy is usually restricted to those with feeding vessels of 3 mm or greater [2].

Typical clinical scenario

Although many patients are asymptomatic, clinical presentations include dyspnea, platypnea (less dyspnea in the supine position – due to decrease in blood flow through the PAVMs in the dependent portions of the lungs in this position), hypoxia, and embolic phenomena (brain abscesses and cerebral ischemia due to right-to-left shunting through the PAVM). Since AVMs can occur in other locations besides the lungs in patients with HHT, epistaxis from nasal mucosal AVMs can also be a presenting symptom.

Differential diagnosis

Hematogenous metastases can sometimes appear to have a feeding vessel, but if carefully examined on CT, particularly with thin-section images, or with reformatted images in the coronal or sagittal planes, it should be apparent that the vessel is not a true feeding vessel. In addition, a draining vein should be demonstrated.

> ### Teaching point
>
> The presence of feeding vessels and draining veins, connected by an aneurysmal sac is diagnostic of pulmonary AVM. When a PAVM is identified, the radiologist should look carefully for others, which would indicate the syndrome of HHT. CT is useful for characterizing these lesions, helping to plan therapy, and for surveillance as well as follow-up.

REFERENCES

1. Gossage JR, Kanj G. Pulmonary arteriovenous malformations. A state of the art review. *Am J Respir Crit Care Med* 1998; **158**: 643–661.
2. Whit RI Jr, Lynch-Nyhan A, Terry P, et al. Pulmonary arteriovenous malformations: techniques and long-term outcome of embolotherapy. *Radiology* 1988; **169**: 663–669.

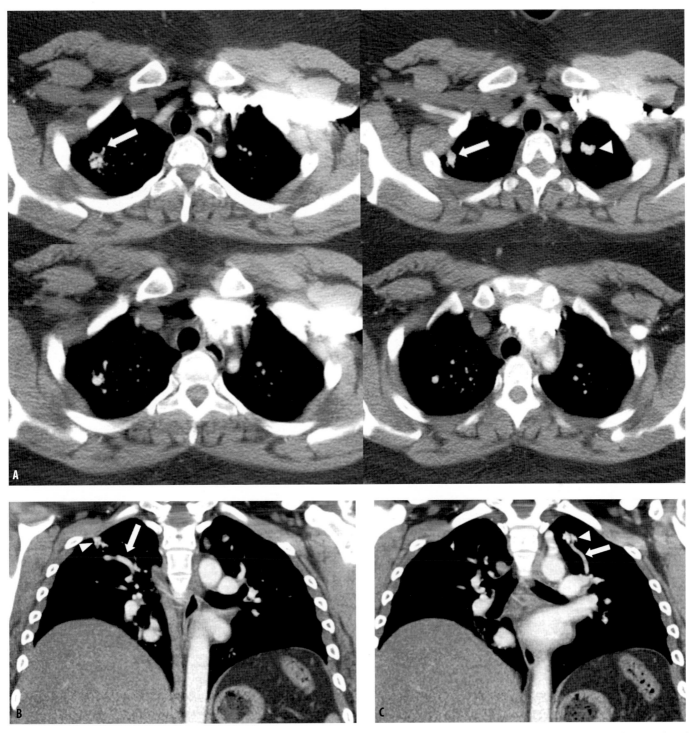

Figure 54.1 A. Axial enhanced CT chest scan shows irregular enhancing nodular densities in both upper lobes (arrow on the right, arrowhead on the left), with feeding arteries and draining veins evident, consistent with AVMs. The multiplicity of lesions suggests Osler-Weber-Rendu syndrome. **B.** Coronal reformatted image from the same study better delineate the feeding and draining vessels: right upper lobe lesion (arrowhead indicates the AVM nidus, and the long white arrow indicates the draining vein). **C.** Left upper lobe lesion (arrowhead indicates the AVM nidus, and the long white arrow indicates the draining vein).

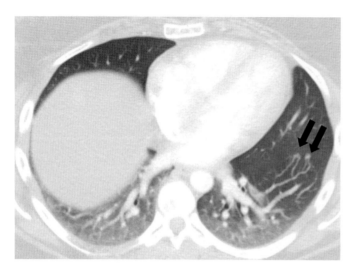

Figure 54.2 Axial lung windows on the same patient as in Figure 54.1 show very tiny AVMs in the left lower lobe (arrows), demonstrating feeding and draining vessels.

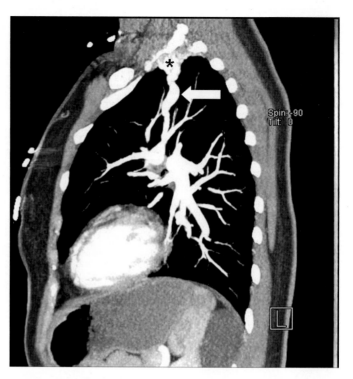

Figure 54.3 Sagittal maximum intensity projection reconstruction image shows a large AVM in the left apex (asterisk) with a large draining vein (arrow).

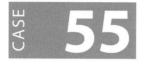
55 Pulmonary artery sarcoma

Anne-Marie Sykes

Imaging description

Primary pulmonary artery sarcomas are rare malignancies, most often "undifferentiated spindle cell sarcomas" or leiomyosarcomas, and are of unknown etiology. They usually arise from the dorsal area of the pulmonary trunk (although they can arise from the right or left pulmonary arteries, pulmonary outflow tract, or pulmonary valve) and are identified on enhanced CT chest as a low-attenuation filling defect (typically solitary) within the lumen of the pulmonary artery. This filling defect may occupy the entire luminal diameter of the artery, may expand the artery, (Figures 55.1–55.3) or may extend through the artery wall [1]. Contrast-enhancement within the tumor has been described, but is not commonly evident on CT [2].

Importance

Because of its rarity and similar imaging appearance to pulmonary embolism, this tumor is often mistaken for pulmonary embolism, resulting in inappropriate therapy such as prolonged anticoagulation or thrombolysis, as well as a delay in accurate diagnosis. Delay in diagnosis results in a generally poor prognosis [3].

Typical clinical scenario

Clinical symptoms of pulmonary artery sarcoma are similar to chronic PE [4] (dyspnea, shortness of breath on exertion). Other symptoms and signs may include weight loss, fever, and anemia. Lack of response to anticoagulation should raise the suspicion of a process other than pulmonary embolism.

Differential diagnosis

The main differential diagnosis is pulmonary embolism. Other diagnostic considerations include intravascular tumor metastases and secondary tumor involvement (direct invasion of the pulmonary artery by central lung cancers), which have different therapeutic options.

Teaching point

Although pulmonary artery sarcoma is a rare disease, the diagnosis and appropriate treatment may be delayed as it is frequently mistaken for pulmonary embolism. Pulmonary artery sarcoma should be considered when the clinical scenario does not fit with pulmonary embolism, when there is only a solitary central lesion, or when there is a lack of response to anticoagulation therapy.

REFERENCES

1. Yi CA, Lee KS, Choe YH, et al. Computed tomography in pulmonary artery sarcoma: distinguishing features from pulmonary embolic disease *J Comput Assist Tomogr* 2004; **28**(1) 34–39.
2. Cox JE, Chiles C, Aquino SL, et al. Pulmonary artery sarcoma: a review of clinical and radiologic features. *J Comput Assist Tomogr* 1997; **21**: 750–755.
3. Kim HK, Choi YS, Kim K, et al. Surgical treatment for pulmonary artery sarcoma *Eur J Cardio Thorac Surg* 2008; **33**: 712–716.
4. Kerr KM. Pulmonary artery sarcoma masquerading as chronic thromboembolic pulmonary hypertension. *Nat Clini Pract Cardiovasc Med* 2005; **2**: 108–112.

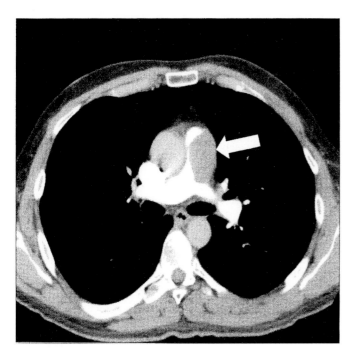

Figure 55.1 Large filling defect in the main pulmonary artery (arrow). Note that it appears somewhat expansile.

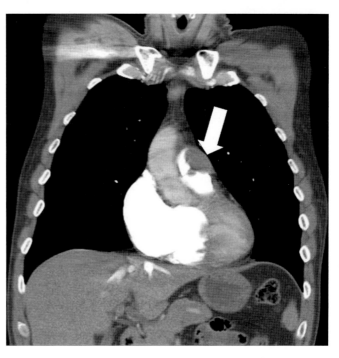

Figure 55.2 Coronal image of the same patient as in Figure 55.1. The "mass" can be seen to be more irregular, and appears to extend beyond the lumen of the pulmonary artery (arrow).

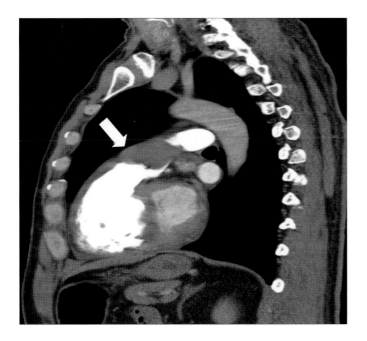

Figure 55.3 Sagittal image of the same patient as in Figure 55.1. Extension beyond the pulmonary artery lumen is even better demonstrated (arrow).

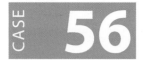

Intravascular tumor emboli

Anne-Marie Sykes

Imaging description

There are two forms of intravascular tumor emboli:

1. Focally dilated and beaded pulmonary arteries on CT [1], resulting from clumps of tumor cells that become lodged within the lumen of small pulmonary arteries, and result in obstruction of the arteries, similar to bland thromboemboli (Figure 56.1).
2. Tree-in-bud pattern on high-resolution CT (representing prominence of otherwise inconspicuous small peripheral pulmonary arteries), resulting from either minute tumor emboli causing prominent fibrocellular proliferation of the intima with resulting thrombosis and luminal obliteration (thrombotic microangiopathy) [2], or filling of the centrilobular arteries with tumor cells themselves (Figures 56.2 and 56.3).

Importance

Pulmonary intravascular tumor emboli are seen in up to 26% of autopsies [3] but are much less frequently identified prior to death. Common extrapulmonary malignancies that cause pulmonary tumor emboli include hepatocellular, breast, renal, stomach and prostate, and choriocarcinoma [4]. Occasionally, this can be the presenting feature of neoplastic disease. The diagnosis of pulmonary endovascular choriocarcinoma in young female patients is of particular importance because it is potentially curable with chemotherapy [5].

Typical clinical scenario

Patients usually present with dyspnea, either acutely or over several weeks. They may also have pleuritic chest pain, cough, and hemoptysis. They may show signs of hypoxia and pulmonary hypertension [6]. The mortality is very high.

Differential diagnosis

The main differential diagnosis is bland pulmonary thromboembolic disease.

Teaching point

Consider intravascular tumor emboli if the affected vessels are beaded in appearance. In the appropriate clinical setting, this diagnosis can also be considered when a tree-in-bud pattern is seen on high-resolution CT.

REFERENCES

1. Franquet T, Gimenez A, Prats R, Rodriguez-Arias JM, Rodriguez C. Thrombotic microangiopathy of pulmonary tumors: a vascular cause of tree-in-bud pattern on CT. *AJR Am J Roentgenol* 2002; **179**: 897–899.
2. Shepard JA, Moore EH, Templeton PA, McLoud TC. Pulmonary intravascular tumor emboli: dilated and beaded peripheral pulmonary arteries at CT. *Radiology* 1993; **187**: 797–801.
3. Schriner RW, Ryu JH, Edwards WD. Microscopic pulmonary tumor embolism causing subacute cor pulmonale: a difficult antemortem diagnosis. *Mayo Clin Proc* 1991; **66**: 143–148.
4. Han D, Lee KS, Franquet T, et al. Thrombotic and nonthrombotic pulmonary arterial embolism: spectrum of imaging findings. *Radiographics* 2003; **23**: 1521–1539.
5. Seckl MJ, Rustin GJ, Newlands Es, Guryther SJ, Bomanji J. Pulmonary embolism, pulmonary hypertension, and choriocarcinoma. *Lancet* 1991; **338**: 1313–1315.
6. Pinckard JK, Wick MR. Tumor-related thrombotic pulmonary microangiopathy: review of pathologic findings and pathophysiologic mechanisms. *Ann Diagn Pathol* 2000; **4**: 154–157.

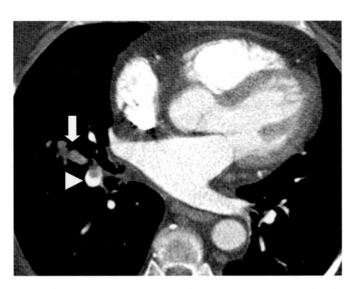

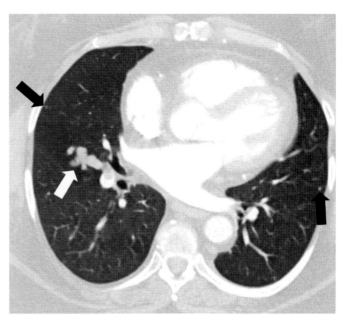

Figure 56.1 Intravascular tumor emboli. Intravascular filling defect in right lower lobe pulmonary artery (arrow) mimics pulmonary thromboembolism. Nodularity of "thrombus" just distally, should raise the suspicion for tumor emboli (arrowhead).

Figure 56.2 Intravascular tumor emboli. Note nodularity and beading of the vessels due to tumor emboli (white arrow). Small pulmonary nodules due to metastases (black arrows) are also evident.

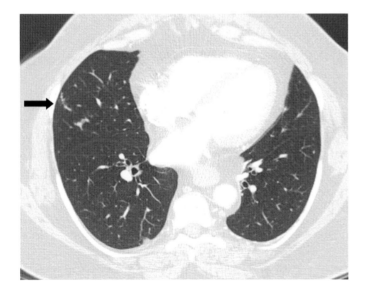

Figure 56.3 Intravascular tumor emboli. Beading of peripherally affected arteries (black arrow).

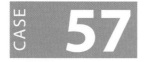

Pulmonary veno-occlusive disease

Anne-Marie Sykes

Imaging description

Pulmonary veno-occlusive disease (PVOD) is considered a cause of pulmonary hypertension that preferentially affects the post-capillary pulmonary vasculature. The pathologic hallmark of PVOD is the extensive and diffuse occlusion of pulmonary veins by fibrous tissue. The imaging findings are a result of this fibrotic occlusion. Pulmonary and pleural lymphatics are dilated. The most consistent parenchymal change is thickening of the interlobular septa due to interstitial edema and deposition of collagen fibers along the septa [1]. On CT chest this is seen as peripheral interlobular septal thickening (Figures 57.1 and 57.2) Alveolar capillaries may become engorged and tortuous, and may resemble pulmonary capillary hemangiomatosis. On CT this is manifested by ground-glass opacities, predominately centrilobular ground-glass nodular opacities [2] (Figures 57.2 and 57.3). Other associated findings at CT include pleural effusions, pericardial effusions, enlarged central pulmonary arteries, normal central pulmonary vein and left atrium size, and mediastinal adenopathy.

Importance

The clinical presentation of PVOD (dyspnea, fatigue) is similar to primary pulmonary hypertension (PPH), but the treatments for PPH (vasodilator therapies) can be harmful and occasionally fatal in patients with PVOD, as they can induce fulminant pulmonary edema [2].

Typical clinical scenario

Most patients with PVOD present with progressive dyspnea upon exertion. Right-sided heart failure may be initially suspected, owing to edema, jugular venous distension, and hypoxemia; however, the chest radiograph findings of bilateral pulmonary infiltrates and Kerley B lines suggest left-sided heart failure. When these patients are evaluated using echocardiography or right-sided heart catheterization, the diagnosis of pulmonary hypertension is confirmed, but the pulmonary wedge pressures are within normal limits. In summary, PVOD

is currently recognized based on one of two sets of findings, as follows:

- The patient is diagnosed with pulmonary arterial hypertension, but a review of the chest radiograph and CT scan raises the suggestion of pulmonary edema.
- The patient is diagnosed with suspected pulmonary edema, but echocardiography or right-sided heart catheterization reveals pulmonary hypertension [3].

Differential diagnosis

Clinically the main differential diagnosis is primary pulmonary hypertension. On CT chest the differential considerations relate to what imaging findings predominate. In early stages, if there is predominately centrilobular ground-glass nodularity, the CT findings may mimic hypersensitivity pneumonitis (HSP), although enlarged central pulmonary arteries are not a feature of HSP. When interlobular septal thickening and pleural effusions predominate, a misdiagnosis of pulmonary edema may be made.

> ## Teaching point
>
> PVOD is an uncommon but important cause of pulmonary hypertension. Although the imaging findings are not pathognomonic and other disease entities may be entertained based on imaging alone, the correlation of the imaging findings with physical examination and right-sided heart catheterization or echocardiography should allow the correct diagnosis to be suggested.

REFERENCES

1. Mandel J, Mark EJ, Hales CA. Pulmonary veno-occlusive disease *Am J Respir Crit Care Med* 2000; **162**(5): 1964–1973.
2. Resten A, Maitre S, Humbert M, et al. Pulmonary hypertension: CT of the chest in pulmonary veno-occlusive disease *AJR Am J Roentgenol* 2004; **183**: 65–70.
3. Hakim AA, Alam S. *Pulmonary veno-occlusive disease eMedicine* January 14, 2009.

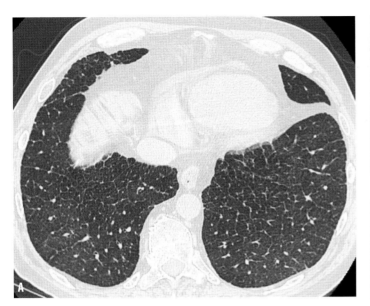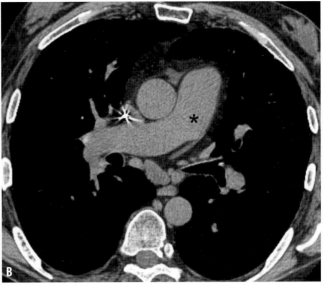

Figure 57.1 Pulmonary veno-occlusive disease with **A.** interlobular septal thickening as the predominant finding on lung windows and **B.** enlargement of the central pulmonary arteries (asterisk).

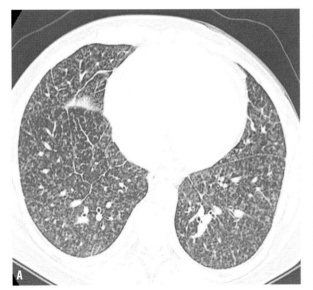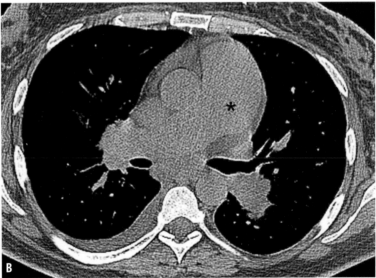

Figure 57.2 Pulmonary veno-occlusive disease with **A.** interlobular septal thickening and centrilobular ground-glass attenuation nodules on the lung windows and **B.** enlargement of the central pulmonary arteries (asterisk), right pleural effusion, and pericardial effusion on the mediastinal windows.

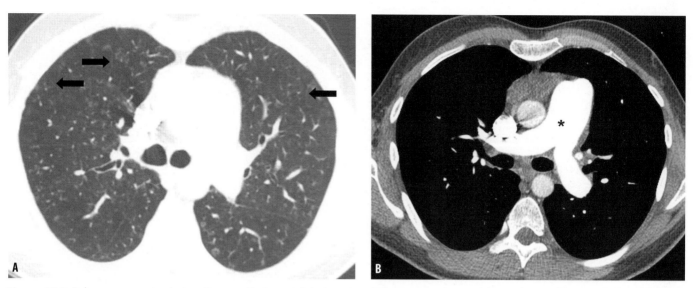

Figure 57.3 Pulmonary veno-occlusive disease with **A.** centrilobular ground-glass attenuation nodules as the predominate finding on lung windows although there are a few thickened interlobular septa (arrows). **B.** Mediastinal windows shows enlargement of the central pulmonary arteries (asterisk).

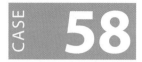

CASE 58

Persistent left SVC

John Hildebrandt and Thomas Hartman

Imaging description

A persistent left superior vena cava (PLSVC) is present in 0.3% of a healthy population and approximately 4.4% of patients with congenital heart disease [1]. A left brachiocephalic vein is either very small or absent in 65% of patients with PLSVC [2]. In approximately 10% of cases with a PLSVC, the right SVC will be absent. The CT imaging of a PLSVC is the same in all cases [2, 3], but the presence of the left brachiocephalic vein and right SVC will be variable. A PLSVC is seen as a tubular structure running along the left side of the mediastinum from the region of the origin of the left brachiocephalic vein inferiorly. In approximately 90% of cases, the PLSVC will drain into the coronary sinus (Figures 58.1–58.3). In the other 10%, the PLSVC will drain into the left atrium (Figure 58.4). Absence of the left brachiocephalic vein results in the left upper body veins draining by way of the PLSVC.

Importance

When a PLSVC is found on CT imaging, it is important to identify whether it drains into the coronary sinus or the left atrium since those that drain into the left atrium will result in a right-to-left shunt.

It is also important to identify whether the left brachiocephalic vein and/or right SVC are present. Absence of the left brachiocephalic vein may have implications for surgery and for placement of a catheter or cardiac pacemaker via a left-sided approach as it will always follow the course of the left SVC. Absence of the right SVC has a higher incidence of associated congenital anomalies [4].

Technical clinical scenario

In cases where a PLSVC and a right SVC are present with or without a left brachiocephalic vein, they are typically asymptomatic and discovered incidentally during imaging for another indication. Occasionally, they may be discovered at the time of imaging for placement of a left-sided catheter

when the catheter is seen to run inferiorly along the left side of the mediastinum.

The minority of cases where the right SVC is absent may be discovered earlier because of associated congenital anomalies such as atrial septal defect, bicuspid aortic valve, and coarctation [4].

Finally, the minority of cases where the PLSVC drains into the left atrium instead of the coronary sinus are often discovered earlier because of the right-to-left shunt created by the drainage into the left atrium which can result in paradoxical embolism.

Differential diagnosis

The differential diagnosis includes partial anomalous pulmonary venous drainage of the left upper lobe and an enlarged cardiophrenic vein. The diagnosis of PLSVC can be made by tracing the course of the left SVC into the coronary sinus.

Teaching point

A PLSVC is relatively common and is normally asymptomatic and hemodynamically insignificant. However, in a minority of cases, the left SVC can drain into the left atrium resulting in a right-to-left shunt.

REFERENCES

1. Cha EM, Khoury GH. Persistent left superior vena cava. Radiologic and clinical significance. *Radiology* 1972; **103**(2): 375–381.
2. Webb WR, Gamsu G, Speckman JM, et al. Computed tomography demonstration of mediastinal venous anomalies. *AJR Am J Roentgenol* 1982; **139**(1): 157–161.
3. Huggins TJ, Lesar ML, Friedman AC, et al. CT appearance of persistent left superior vena cava. *J Comput Assist Tomogr* 1982; **6**: 294–297.
4. Sarodia B, Stoller J. Persistent left superior vena cava: case report and literature review. *Respir Care* 2000; **45**(4): 411–416.

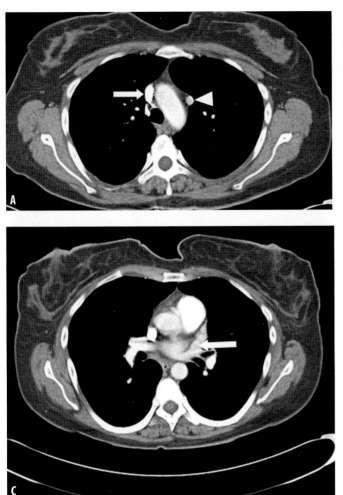

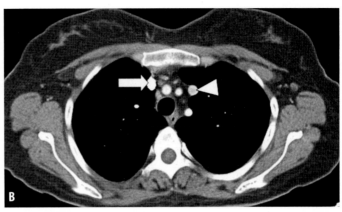

Figure 58.1 A. Contrast-enhanced axial CT at the level of the aortic arch demonstrates the presence of a right (arrow) and left (arrowhead) SVC. B. Contrast-enhanced CT chest in the superior mediastinum shows no left brachiocephalic vein. The right (arrow) and left (arrowhead) SVC are seen instead. C. Contrast-enhanced CT chest shows the left SVC draining into the coronary sinus (arrow).

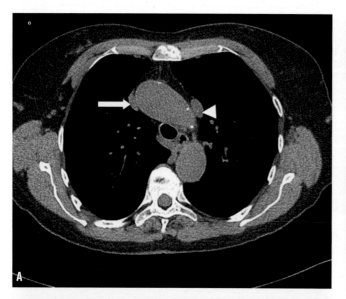

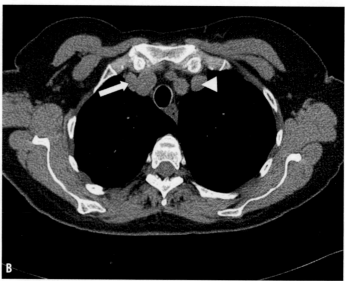

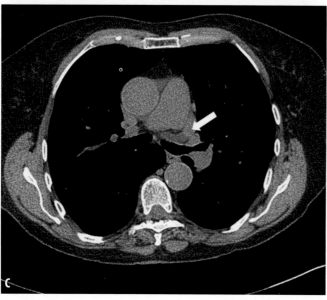

Figure 58.2 A. Axial CT without contrast at the level of the aortic arch demonstrates the presence of a right (arrow) and left (arrowhead) SVC. **B.** Axial CT without contrast in the superior mediastinum shows no left brachiocephalic vein. The right (arrow) and left (arrowhead) SVC are seen instead. **C.** Axial CT without contrast shows the left SVC draining into the coronary sinus (arrow).

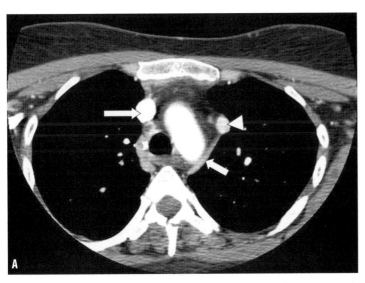
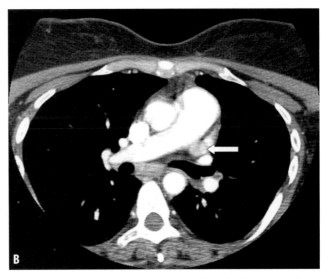

Figure 58.3 **A.** Contrast-enhanced axial CT at the level of the aortic arch demonstrates a right (arrow) and left (arrowhead) SVC. Also note that the left superior intercostal vein (small arrow) is draining into the PLSVC. **B.** Contrast-enhanced CT chest shows the left SVC draining into the coronary sinus (arrow).

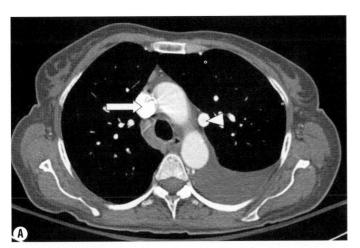
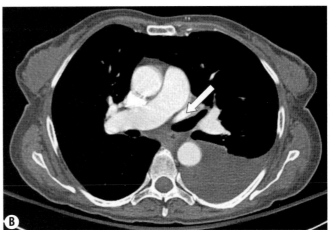
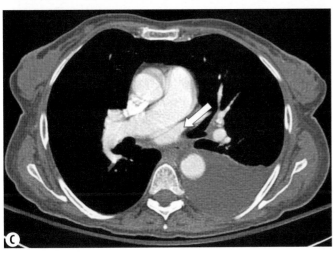

Figure 58.4 **A.** Contrast-enhanced axial CT at the level of the aortic arch demonstrates the presence of a right (arrow) and left (arrowhead) SVC. A left pleural effusion is also present. **B.** Contrast-enhanced axial CT at the level of the right main pulmonary artery shows the PLSVC (arrow) passing posterior to the pulmonary artery. A left pleural effusion is also present. **C.** Contrast-enhanced axial CT at the level of the high left atrium shows the PLSVC (arrow) entering the left atrium. A left pleural effusion is also present.

SVC syndrome

John Hildebrandt

Imaging description

Superior vena cava (SVC) syndrome is most commonly caused by malignancy [1] which usually causes extensive compression. In this setting, a mass or adenopathy will be seen narrowing or obstructing the SVC on CT images (Figure 59.1). If the cause is from intrinsic thrombosis such as from a central line, enlargement of the azygos vein and/or luminal clot within the SVC can be seen on contrast-enhanced CT (Figure 59.2). In addition to the narrowing or occlusion of the SVC, collateral vessels within the chest can be seen and when present the diagnosis of SVC syndrome [2] can be made.

Importance

The most common cause of SVC syndrome is malignancy, with bronchogenic carcinoma being the most common [1]. Of the bronchogenic carcinomas, small cell lung cancer is the most common [3, 4]. The next most commonly associated malignancy is non-Hodgkin's lymphoma. The most common benign cause is fibrosing mediastinitis. It has been estimated that about 78% of causes of SVC syndrome are due to malignant neoplasms and 22% from benign causes such as fibrosing mediastinitis, radiation fibrosis, or indwelling venous catheters [1]. Recognition of SVC syndrome and identification of its cause will help to lead to quicker resolution or improvement in severity of symptoms.

Typical clinical scenario

The clinical signs and symptoms that occur will depend on the degree and speed of obstruction of the SVC and amount of venous collateral formation that develops [5]. Common symptoms include dyspnea and feeling of fullness or congestion in the head. Physical findings include edema and distention of the veins of the face, neck, arms, and upper chest. Generally the diagnosis is made on cross-sectional imaging after presentation of signs and symptoms.

Differential diagnosis

Imaging that demonstrates partial or complete occlusion of the SVC with associated dilated collateral vessels is diagnostic of SVC syndrome.

Teaching point

The majority of cases of SVC syndrome are caused by malignancy and present with classic symptoms and physical findings. Diagnostic imaging should demonstrate narrowing or occlusion of the SVC along with identification of collateral vessels.

REFERENCES

1. Parish JM, Marschke RF Jr, Dines DE, et al. Etiologic considerations in superior vena cava syndrome. *Mayo Clinic Proc* 1981; **56**: 407–413.
2. Kim H-J, Kim HS, Chung SH. CT diagnosis of superior vena cava syndrome: importance of collateral vessels. *Am J Roentegenol* 1993; **161**: 539–542.
3. Chan RH, Dar AR, Yu E, et al. Superior vena cava obstruction in small cell lung cancer. *Int J Radiat Oncol* 1997; **38**: 513–520.
4. Shimm DS, Logue GL, Rigsby LC. Evaluating the superior vena cava syndrome. *JAMA* 1981; **245**: 951–953.
5. Mahagan V, Strimlan V, Ordstrand HS, et al. Benign superior vena cava syndrome. *Chest* 1975; **68**: 32–33.

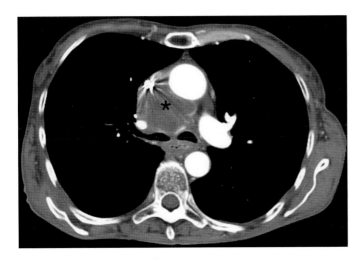

Figure 59.1 Axial enhanced CT image demonstrates large mediastinal soft tissue mass (asterisk) which causes extrinsic compression of the SVC. The patient underwent transbronchial needle aspiration which resulted in the diagnosis of adenocarcinoma of the lung.

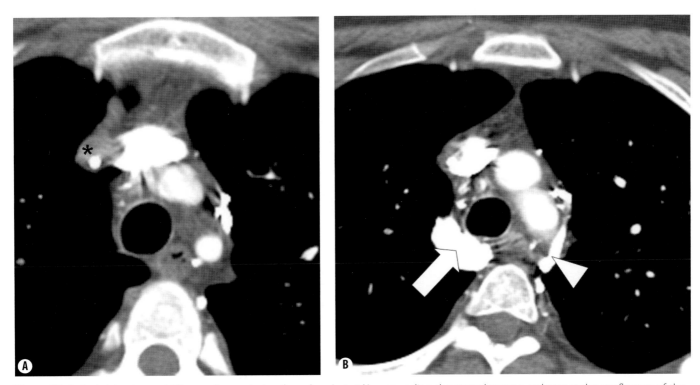

Figure 59.2 **A.** Axial enhanced CT scan demonstrates thrombus (asterisk) surrounding the central venous catheter at the confluence of the innominate veins. **B.** Enhanced axial CT demonstrates dilatation of the azygos vein (arrow) and left superior intercostal vein (arrowhead).

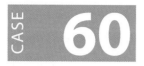

Prominent superior intercostal vein

John Hildebrandt

Imaging description

Distension of the left superior intercostal vein (LSIV) is easily diagnosed on CT or MRI by direction visualization of the vein (Figures 60.1–60.3) and its collateral pathways. CT or MRI can identify the source of its dilatation.

Importance

Prominence of the LSIV is associated with acquired and congenital anomalies. These are described in the clinical scenario section below.

Typical clinical scenario

The presence or absence of clinical signs and symptoms is based on the cause for the prominent LSIV. This is usually a result of distension of the collateral venous system. The LSIV arises from the confluence of the left second through fourth intercostal veins in a left paraspinal location. It courses anteriorly at the T3/T4 level to the left of the aortic arch and drains into the left brachiocephalic vein or persistent left superior vena cava (Figure 60.2) [1, 2]. It has an inferior communication with the accessory hemiazygos vein 75% of the time [3]. This is a collateral pathway to the superior vena cava, hemiazygos, azygos, and lumber veins. Conditions that affect these veins or the left brachiocephalic vein are the source of LSIV distension (Figure 60.3). Congenital causes are azygos continuation of the inferior vena cava, hypoplasia or absence of the left innominate vein and anomalous pulmonary venous return [2]. Acquired causes are superior or inferior vena cava narrowing/obstruction, (Figure 60.1) congestive heart failure, portal hypertension, and Budd-Chiari syndrome [2].

Differential diagnosis

CT or MRI is diagnostic of prominence of the LSIV.

Teaching point

Prominent LSIV is caused by congenital or acquired conditions that affect the collateral venous pathways. Careful evaluation of these pathways on CT or MRI can reveal its etiology.

REFERENCES

1. Hatfield MK, Vyborny CJ, MacMahon H, Chessare JW. Congenital absence of the azygos vein: a cause for "aortic nipple" enlargement. *AJR Am J Roentgenol* 1987; **149**: 273–274.
2. Friedman AC, Chambers E, Sprayregen S. The normal and abnormal left superior intercostal vein. *AJR Am J Roentgenol* 1978; **131**: 599–602.
3. McDonald CJ, Castellino RA, Blank N. The aortic "nipple." The left superior intercostal vein. *Radiology* 1970; **96**: 533–536.

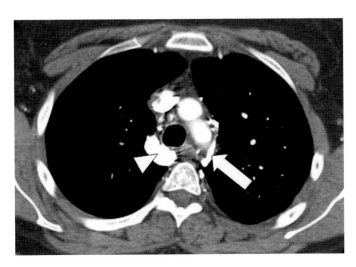

Figure 60.1 CT with contrast shows a prominent left superior intercostal vein along its horizontal course (arrow) and dilatation of the azygos vein (arrowhead) secondary to thrombosis of the superior vena cava (SVC).

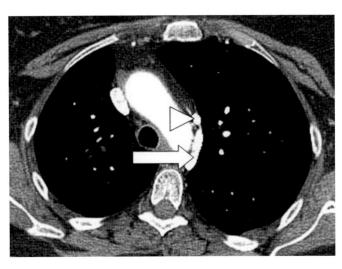

Figure 60.2 CT with contrast shows a prominent left superior intercostal vein (arrow) draining into a persistent left SVC (arrowhead).

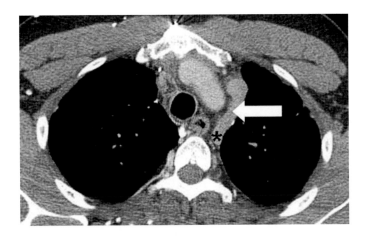

Figure 60.3 CT with contrast shows a prominent left superior intercostal vein (arrow) draining into a dilated accessory hemiazygos vein (asterisk) in a patient with occlusion of the SVC by a teratoma (not seen on this image).

61 Azygos continuation of the IVC

John Hildebrandt

Imaging description

Azygos continuation of the inferior vena cava (IVC) causes dilatation of the azygos and hemiazygos vein. On CT, there is dilatation and tortuosity of the veins as well as infrahepatic interruption of the IVC (Figures 61.1 and 61.2). Recognition of the interruption of the infrahepatic IVC is important to make the correct diagnosis.

Importance

The dilated azygos vein on noncontrast CT can be mistaken for a large azygos lymph node or mass. However, recognition of dilatation of the azygos vein and hemiazygos vein with interruption of the infrahepatic IVC will allow the correct diagnosis.

Typical clinical scenario

Azygos continuation of the IVC has a prevalence of 0.6% [1]. Most of the patients are asymptomatic. However, complications consisting of compression of the right mainstem bronchus [2] and obstruction of the superior vena cava (SVC) [3] can occur.

Differential diagnosis

On noncontrast CT, the dilated azygos vein may be mistaken for right paratracheal adenopathy or mass. Azygos dilatation from other causes such as SVC obstruction should also be considered. However, recognition of the associated findings (dilated azygos and hemiazygos veins with interruption of the intrahepatic IVC) will allow the correct diagnosis.

Teaching point

Azygos continuation of the IVC is one of several etiologies that cause enlargement of the azygos and hemiazygos vein. The CT findings of dilatation of the azygos and hemiazygos veins with interruption of the intrahepatic IVC are diagnostic.

REFERENCES

1. Ginaldi S, Chuang DP, Wallace S. Absence of the hepatic segment of the inferior vena cava with azygos continuation. *J Comput Assist Tomogr* 1980; **4**: 112–114.
2. Mehta M, Towers M. Computed tomography appearance of idiopathic aneurysm of the azygos vein. *Can Assoc Radiol J* 1996; **47**: 288–290.
3. Seebauer L, Präuer HW, Gmeinwieser J, et al. A mediastinal tumor simulated by a sacculated aneurysm of the azygos vein. *Thorac Cardiovasc Surg* 1989; **37**: 112–114.

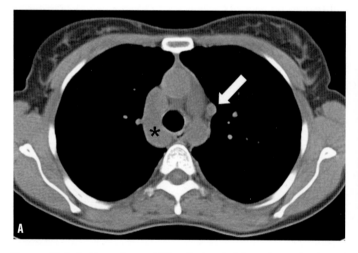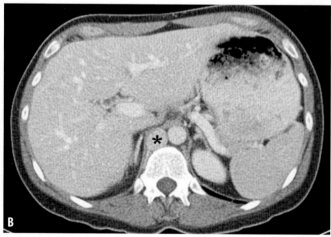

Figure 61.1 A. Nonenhanced CT at the level of the right tracheobronchial angle shows dilatation of the azygos vein (asterisk) and its confluence with the superior vena cava (SVC). A persistent left SVC is also present (arrow). **B.** Abdominal CT with intravenous contrast in the same patient as Figure 61.2A shows dilatation of the azygos vein (asterisk) and absence of the infrahepatic IVC.

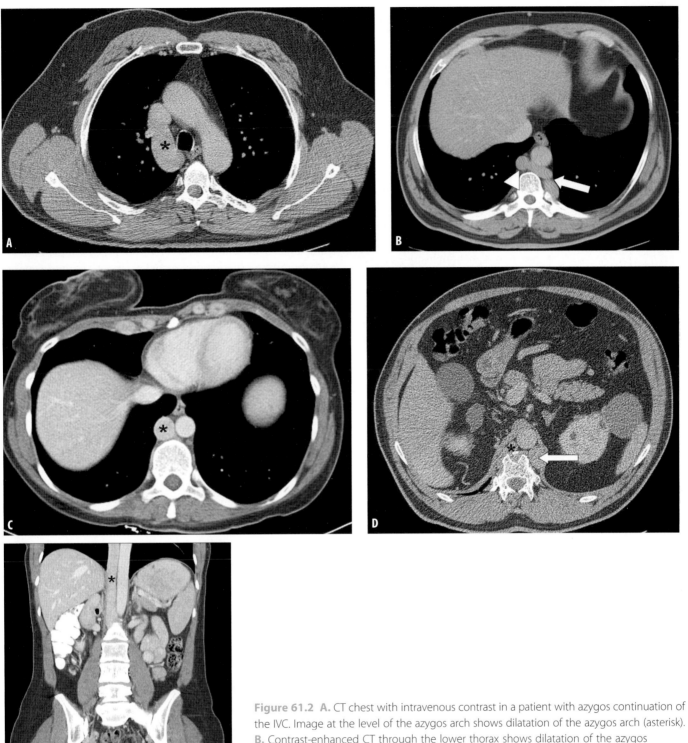

Figure 61.2 **A.** CT chest with intravenous contrast in a patient with azygos continuation of the IVC. Image at the level of the azygos arch shows dilatation of the azygos arch (asterisk). **B.** Contrast-enhanced CT through the lower thorax shows dilatation of the azygos (arrowhead) and the hemiazygos vein (large arrow). **C.** Contrast-enhanced CT through the lower chest shows a dilated azygos vein (asterisk). **D.** Contrast-enhanced CT through the upper abdomen shows a dilated azygos vein (asterisk) and a dilated hemiazygos vein (arrow) with absence of the infrahepatic IVC. **E.** Coronal reconstruction of the abdomen shows a dilated azygos vein (asterisk) to the right of the aorta.

62 Recesses of the pericardium

Rebecca Lindell

Imaging description

The pericardium is composed of two layers: a tough fibrous outer layer, which attaches to the diaphragm, sternum, and costal cartilage, and a thin inner serous layer, which lies adjacent to the heart [1, 2]. The normal pericardium may contain 15 to 50 ml of fluid [1, 2]. On CT and MRI, the normal pericardium appears as a thin linear structure measuring less than 2 mm surrounding the heart but may not be visualized over the left ventricle, where it often becomes very thin [1, 2]. On MRI, it has low signal intensity on both T1- and T2-weighted images and is outlined by high signal intensity mediastinal and subepicardial fat [1, 2]. The pericardium extends superiorly about the main pulmonary artery, ascending aorta, and superior vena cava [3].

The serous layer of the pericardium can be divided into parietal and visceral layers [4]. As the visceral pericardium adheres to the heart and great vessels, the separation from the parietal pericardium creates recesses and sinuses that may be seen on CT or MRI [3, 4]. The transverse sinus is located just above the left atrium and posterior to the ascending aorta and main pulmonary artery (Figure 62.1) [1–3, 5]. The superior reflection of the transverse sinus is known as the superior aortic recess, which has anterior, posterior, and right lateral portions [1, 3]. On CT, the posterior portion lies directly posterior to the ascending aorta at the level of the left pulmonary artery, is of fluid attenuation, and usually has a crescent shape (Figure 62.2) [3, 5]. This recess may extend into the high right paratracheal region (Figure 62.3) [5, 6]. The oblique sinus is the posterior extension of the pericardium and lies posterior to the left atrium and anterior to the esophagus [1–3] (Figure 62.4). Recesses may also arise from the pericardial cavity proper [3]. In particular, recesses may extend along the pulmonary veins (Figure 62.5). There are also smaller pericardial recesses including posterolateral to the superior vena cava and between the inferior vena cava and coronary sinus [4].

Importance

Knowledge of the pericardial anatomy and recesses prevents mistaking them for pathology such as adenopathy, dissection, or cysts.

Typical clinical scenario

Pericardial recesses are normal and may become more prominent with pericardial effusion.

Differential diagnosis

Depending upon the location, pericardial sinuses and recesses may be mistaken for adenopathy, aortic dissection, or

mediastinal cysts [1, 2, 7]. Familiarity with the location of pericardial recesses, as well as their usual configuration and attenuation should prevent misdiagnosis.

For example, the posterior portion of the superior aortic recess can be mistaken for a pre-carinal lymph node (Figure 62.6). Lymph nodes are of soft tissue attenuation and typically are separated from the aorta by mediastinal fat. The superior aortic recess may extend into the high right paratracheal region and may be mistaken for adenopathy or a bronchogenic cyst [5, 6]. Another example is that fluid in the anterior portion of the superior pericardial recess can be mistaken for aortic dissection or an anterior mediastinal cyst (Figures 62.7 and 62.8) [7]. In addition, the oblique sinus must be distinguished from subcarinal adenopathy, a bronchogenic cyst, or an esophageal lesion [1–3]. Pulmonic vein recesses can be mistaken for bronchopulmonary lymph nodes [3]. In all cases, reformatted images may be helpful to see the connection of the area in question to the pericardial space (Figure 62.3).

Teaching point

Pericardial recesses are normal and may become prominent with pericardial effusion. Knowledge of their location and imaging appearance is essential to avoid mistaking them for adenopathy, dissection, or mediastinal cysts.

REFERENCES
1. Lopez Costa I, Bhalla S. Computed tomography and magnetic resonance imaging of the pericardium. *Semin Roentgenol* 2008; **43**(3): 234–245.
2. Oyama N, Oyama N, Kumuro K, et al. Computed tomography and magnetic resonance imaging of the pericardium: anatomy and pathology. *Magn Reson Med Sci* 2004; **3**: 145–152.
3. Broderick LS, Brooks GN, Kuhlman JE. Anatomic pitfalls of the heart and pericardium. *Radiographics* 2005; **25**: 441–453.
4. Levy-Ravetch M, Auh YH, Rubenstein WA, Whalen JP, Kazam E. CT of the pericardial recesses. *AJR Am J Roentgenol* 1985; **144**: 707–714.
5. Truong MT, Erasmus JJ, Gladish GW, et al. Anatomy of pericardial recesses on multidetector CT: implications for oncologic imaging. *AJR Am J Roentgenol* 2003; **181**: 1109–1113.
6. Choi YW, McAdams HP, Jeon SC, Seo HS, Hahm CK. The "high-riding" superior pericardial recess: CT findings. *AJR Am J Roentgenol* 2000; **175**: 1025–1028
7. Winer-Muram HT, Gold RE. Effusion in the superior pericardial recess simulating a mediastinal mass. *AJR Am J Roentgenol* 1990; **154**: 69–71.

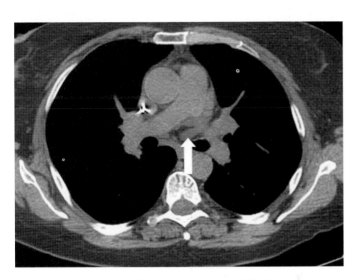

Figure 62.1 Axial image from an unenhanced CT chest shows the transverse sinus (arrow) situated behind the main pulmonary artery and above the left atrium.

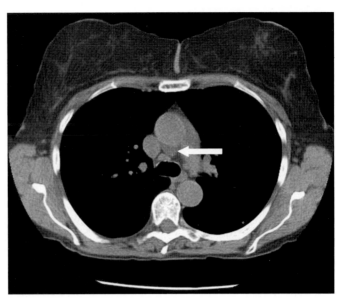

Figure 62.2 Axial image from a noncontrast CT chest shows fluid attenuation posterior to the ascending aorta (arrow). This is the superior pericardial recess and should not be mistaken for adenopathy.

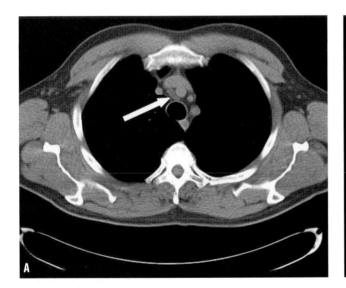

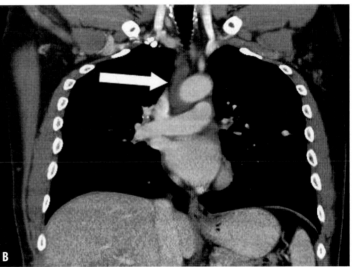

Figure 62.3 A. Axial image from a noncontrast CT chest shows a fluid attenuation oval opacity anterior to the trachea (arrow).
B. Contrast-enhanced coronal reconstruction shows extension from the pericardium (arrow), confirming that the structure is consistent with a high-riding pericardial recess.

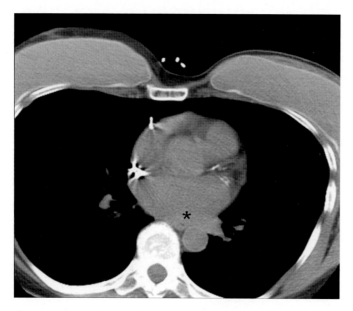

Figure 62.4 Axial image from a nonenhanced CT chest shows a tiny amount of fluid attenuation posterior to the left atrium (asterisk), compatible with the oblique sinus.

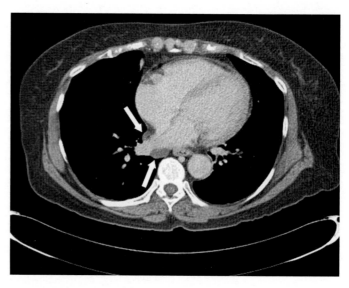

Figure 62.5 Axial image from a contrasted enhanced chest CT shows prominent fluid attenuation (arrows) along the right inferior pulmonary vein. This is consistent with a normal but prominent pericardial recess.

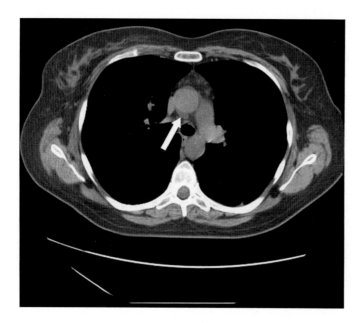

Figure 62.6 Axial image from a noncontrast CT chest shows crescentoid fluid attenuation posterior to the ascending aorta (arrow) without intervening mediastinal fat. This is the superior pericardial recess and should not be mistaken for adenopathy.

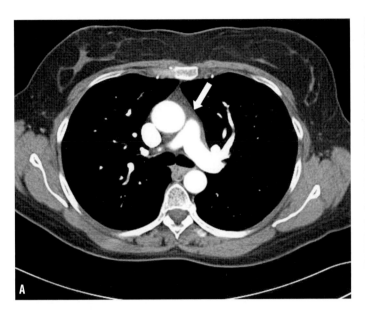

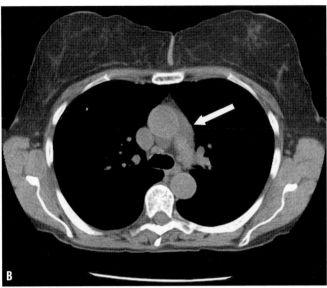

Figure 62.7 A. Axial image from a contrast-enhanced CT chest shows a small triangular-shaped fluid attenuation (arrow) between the ascending aorta and pulmonary trunk. This is the anterior portion of the superior pericardial recess and, when distended, should not be mistaken for aortic dissection. **B.** Axial image from a noncontrast CT chest in a different patient shows a more distended but normal anterior portion of the superior pericardial recess (arrow).

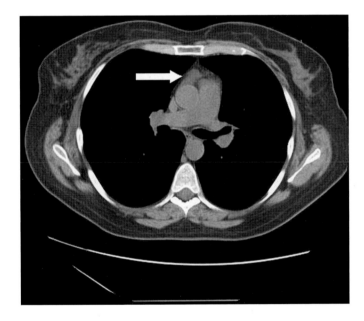

Figure 62.8 Axial image from a nonenhanced CT chest in a woman with a tiny pericardial effusion shows fluid attenuation (arrow) anterior to the ascending aorta. This is the anterior portion of the superior pericardial recess and, when distended, should not be mistaken for aortic dissection or anterior mediastinal cyst.

63 Pericardial effusion

Rebecca Lindell and Thomas Hartman

Imaging description

Pericardial effusion is caused by the obstruction of the lymphatic or venous drainage from the heart [1]. Accumulation of pericardial fluid above 50 ml is abnormal, which corresponds to 4 mm thickness of the pericardium on cross-sectional imaging [2, 3] (Figure 63.1). Simple effusions tend to have the attenuation of water on CT (<10 HU) (Figures 63.2 and 63.3), while exudative (20–60 HU) or hemorrhagic (60–80 HU) effusions have attenuation values greater than that of water [2, 4]. Pericardial effusions accompanied by pericardial thickening are suggestive of inflammatory pericarditis [4]. MRI can be helpful in characterizing pericardial effusions [3–5] (Figure 63.4). Signal characteristics may help distinguish pericardial fluid from thickening or may distinguish between simple and exudative or hemorrhagic transudative effusions. Simple effusions have no or very little T1-weighted signal intensity, while exudative or hemorrhagic effusions often are medium or high signal intensity on T1 sequences [3–5].

Importance

Pericardial effusions are often asymptomatic but large effusions may be symptomatic and, therefore, are important to identify in order to alert the clinician. Occasionally the cause of a pericardial effusion can be identified on cross-sectional imaging, especially in cases of hemopericardium.

Typical clinical scenario

Pericardial effusions are caused by a wide variety of systemic or cardiac diseases, such as infectious or idiopathic pericarditis, postinfarction syndrome, neoplasm, uremia, trauma, radiation therapy, collagen vascular disease, and AIDS [3–6].

Differential diagnosis

A pericardial effusion surrounding the heart is usually easy to diagnose on CT. However, if it is loculated it may be confused with a pericardial cyst. The attenuation of a pericardial effusion may help to identify the cause. An effusion with an attenuation higher than that of water narrows the differential to trauma, malignancy, purulent exudate, or hypothyroidism-associated effusion [6]. Effusions associated with nodularity or irregular thickening can be seen in pericardial neoplastic involvement [6]. Small pericardial effusions may be difficult to distinguish from mild pericardial thickening [6].

Teaching point

The attenuation of a pericardial effusion as well as any associated thickening or nodularity may be helpful in identifying its cause. Some causes of pericardial effusions, such as aortic dissection, may be directly visualized. It may be difficult to distinguish tiny pericardial effusions from mild pericardial thickening.

REFERENCES

1. Wang ZJ, Reddy GP, Gotway MB, et al. CT and MR imaging of pericardial disease. *Radiographics* 2003; **23**: S167–S180.
2. Lopez Costa I, Bhalla S. Computed tomography and magnetic resonance imaging of the pericardium. *Semin Roentgenol* 2008; **43**(3): 234–245.
3. Glockner JF. Imaging of pericardial disease. *Magn Reson Imaging Clin N Am* 2003; **11**: 149–162.
4. Olson MC, Posniak HV, McDonald V, et al. Computed tomography and magnetic resonance imaging of the pericardium. *Radiographics* 1989; **9**: 633–649.
5. Breen JF. Imaging of the pericardium. *J Thorac Imaging* 2001; **16**: 47–54.
6. Kim JS, Kim HH, Yoon Y. Imaging of pericardial diseases. *Clin Radiol* 2007; **62**(7): 626–631.

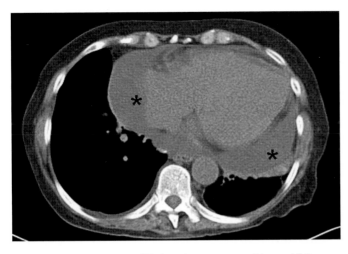

Figure 63.1 Noncontrast CT chest in a woman with renal failure shows a large fluid attenuation collection surrounding the heart most marked laterally (asterisks), compatible with a large pericardial effusion.

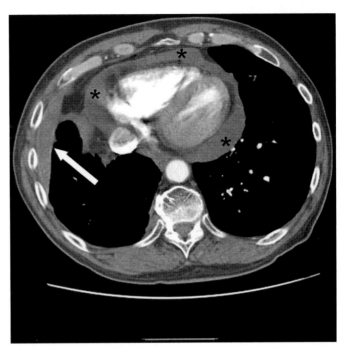

Figure 63.2 Enhanced CT chest axial image in a patient being treated for unresectable lung cancer shows a small pericardial effusion (asterisks) and a small loculated pleural effusion in the right chest (arrow).

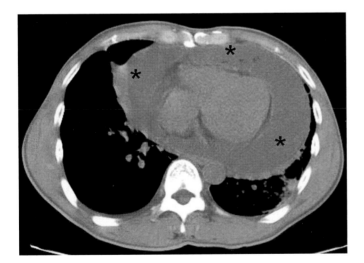

Figure 63.3 Noncontrast CT chest in a man with a history of prior tuberculosis shows a large pericardial effusion (asterisks). The patient underwent a pericardial windows procedure and cultures showed tuberculous pericarditis.

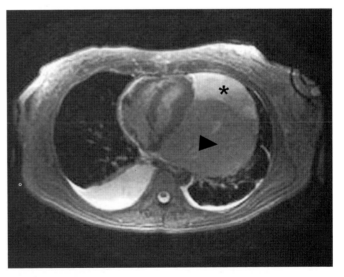

Figure 63.4 Steady-state free precession MRI in a woman showing a large pericardial mass (arrowhead) and pericardial effusion (asterisk). Also note bilateral pleural effusions.

Imaging description

Pericardial cysts are congenital lesions that are formed when a portion of the pericardium is pinched off during early development. Pericardial cysts can occur anywhere within the mediastinum, but are most common in the cardiophrenic angles. On CT, pericardial cysts typically have thin to undetectable walls without septation (Figure 64.1). There is no enhancement following contrast administration [1–3] (Figures 64.2 and 64.3). The attenuation of pericardial cysts is usually that of water although rarely they can be higher attenuation. In those cases, MRI is often helpful in determining the fluid nature of the lesion. The cysts usually have low to intermediate signal intensity on T1-weighted imaging although in cases with proteinaceous material in the cyst there may be high signal on T1-weighted imaging. The cysts have homogeneous high signal intensity on T2-weighted imaging [1–3].

Importance

Recognition of the fluid attenuation of the pericardial mass allows the exclusion of pericardial or mediastinal neoplasms. Since these are typically asymptomatic, no further workup or treatment is necessary.

Differential diagnosis

When pericardial cysts are present in the cardiophrenic angles, the appearance and location are diagnostic. However, pericardial cysts can occur in other locations in the mediastinum and in those instances a pericardial cyst can be difficult to distinguish from a bronchogenic cyst or a thymic cyst.

Teaching point

A fluid attenuation mass with thin or imperceptible walls in the cardiophrenic angles on CT or MRI should be a pericardial cyst. If the patient is asymptomatic, no further workup or treatment is necessary.

REFERENCES
1. Wang ZJ, Reddy GP, Gotway MB, et al. CT and MR imaging of pericardial disease. *Radiographics* 2003; **23** Spec No: S167–S180.
2. Olson MC, Posniak HV, McDonald V, Wisniewski R, Moncada R. Computed tomography and magnetic resonance imaging of the pericardium. *Radiographics* 1989; **9**: 633–649.
3. Reinmuller R, Groll R, Lipton MJ. CT and MR imaging of pericardial disease. *Radiol Clin North Am* 2004; **42**: 587–601.

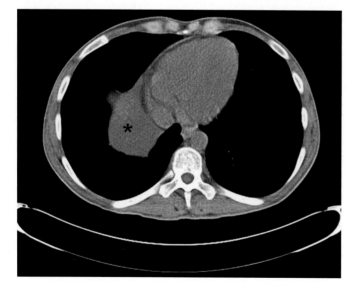

Figure 64.1 CT chest without contrast shows a fluid attenuation mass (asterisk) arising from the right side of the mediastinum. There is no perceptible wall and the mass is in continuity with the pericardium. Findings are typical of a pericardial cyst.

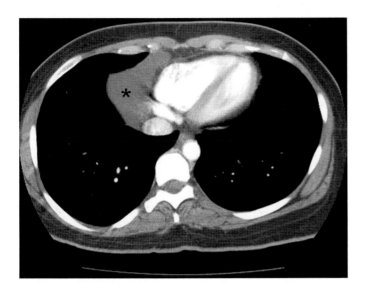

Figure 64.2 CT chest with contrast shows a pericardial cyst in the right cardiophrenic angle (asterisk). The wall of the cyst is imperceptible and there is no enhancement.

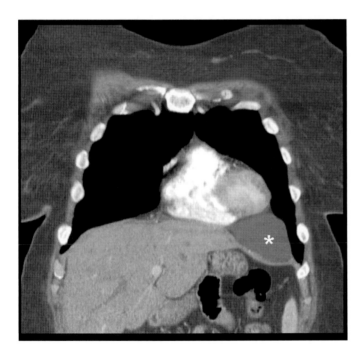

Figure 64.3 Coronal reconstruction of a CT chest with contrast shows a pericardial cyst in the left cardiophrenic angle (asterisk).

Partial or complete absence of the pericardium

Rebecca Lindell

Imaging description

Pericardial defects may be congenital, posttraumatic, or postsurgical [1]. Congenital pericardial defects are rare and most often occur on the left [1–3]. Extent of congenital pericardial absence is variable and complete absence of the entire pericardium is exceptionally rare [2]. In fact, the term "complete absence" is at times used to refer to large partial defects that result in cardiac displacement into the left pleural cavity [2]. Congenital defects are attributed to premature atrophy of the left common cardinal vein, which cuts off blood supply to the developing pericardium [2, 3]. On CT and MRI, partial absence of the pericardium may be small enough that normal pericardial position is maintained but the heart is at risk of herniation through the defect with or without incarceration. Large partial defects and complete absence of the pericardium show leftward and/or posterior displacement of the heart on CT and MRI [1, 4, 5] (Figures 65.1 and 65.2). Partial or complete defects may allow interposition of lung tissue between the aorta and the main pulmonary artery or between the base of the heart and the diaphragm, which can help to make the diagnosis on imaging [1, 3–5]. A portion of the heart, such as the left atrium, may bulge through the defect on imaging [1]. The actual pericardial defect may be directly visualized on CT or MRI, although normal intact pericardium may not be readily visualized over the left atrial appendage or left ventricle [4].

Importance

Partial absence of the pericardium occurs more frequently than complete absence and has a higher risk for complications [3, 4]. Specifically, patients with partial absence of the pericardium are at risk of herniation and entrapment of the myocardium or cardiac chamber, especially the left atrial appendage [1, 3, 5]. This is a rare but important complication [4].

Typical clinical scenario

Patients are most often asymptomatic. Patients may be symptomatic from associated congenital abnormalities such as atrial septal defect, patent ductus arteriosus, mitral valve stenosis, or tetralogy of Fallot [1, 3]. When herniation or entrapment of the heart or an appendage occurs, angina, syncope, dysrhythmia, or sudden death may occur [3].

Differential diagnosis

It is important to note that an intact normal pericardium often is not visualized over the left atrial appendage and left ventricle, hence lack of visualization of the pericardium on CT or MRI is not sufficient for diagnosis [4]. Levoposition of the heart may also be seen with other cardiac conditions such as atrial septal defect, pulmonary valve stenosis, mitral valve disease, and cor pulmonale with right ventricular dilatation [4]. Identification of lung tissue interposition between the aorta and main pulmonary artery or base of the heart and diaphragm is a strong indication of a pericardial defect and is not present in these other entities [1, 3–5].

Teaching point

Pericardial defects are rare and the extent of the defect may vary. Large defects tend to be asymptomatic but more often have abnormal imaging findings such as leftward and/or posterior rotation of the heart as well as interposition of lung tissue between the aorta and main pulmonary artery or heart base and diaphragm. Small defects may have normal imaging but these patients are at risk for herniation and entrapment of the heart, which is rare but can be fatal.

REFERENCES

1. Wang ZJ, Reddy GP, Gotway MB, et al. CT and MR imaging of pericardial disease. *Radiographics* 2003; **23**: S167–S180.
2. Tan RS, Partridge J, Ilsley C, Mohiaddin R. Familial complete congenital absence of the pericardium. *Clin Radiol* 2007; **62**(1): 85–87.
3. Kim JS, Kim HH, Yoon Y. Imaging of pericardial diseases. *Clin Radiol* 2007; **62**(7): 626–631.
4. Lopez Costa I, Bhalla S. Computed tomography and magnetic resonance imaging of the pericardium. *Semin Roentgenol* 2008; **43**(3): 234–245.
5. Baim RS, MacDonald IL, Wise DJ, Lenkei SC. Computed tomography of absent left pericardium. *Radiology* 1980; **135**: 127–128.

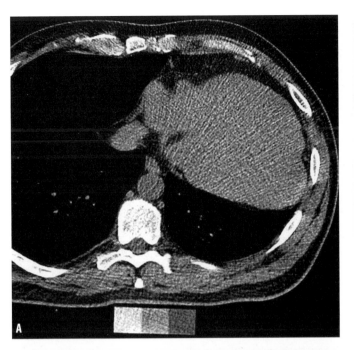

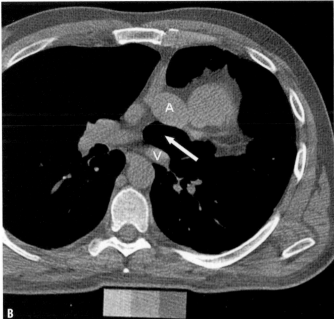

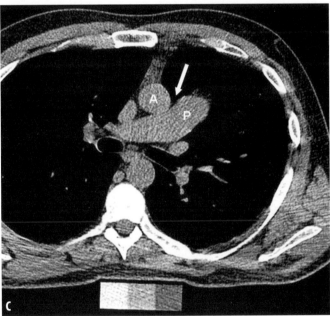

Figure 65.1 A. Axial noncontrast CT chest shows large left pericardial defect and rotation of the heart towards the left. **B.** Axial noncontrast CT chest shows lung tissue abnormally interposed between the ascending aorta (A) and pulmonary vein (V) (arrow). **C.** Axial noncontrast CT chest image shows lung tissue interposed between the ascending aorta (A) and main pulmonary artery (P) (arrow).

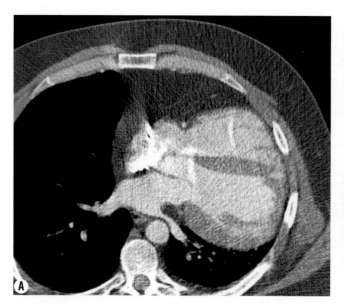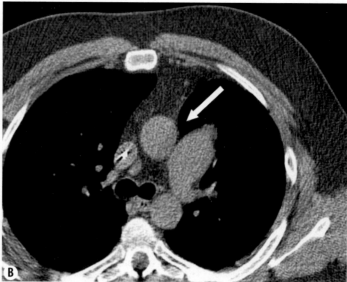

Figure 65.2 A. Axial cardiac CT with intravenous contrast shows large left pericardial defect and rotation of the heart leftward and posteriorly. A pacemaker is present. **B.** Axial noncontrast cardiac CT image at the level of the main pulmonary artery shows interposition of lung tissue between the aorta and main pulmonary artery (arrow).

Pleural lipoma

Rebecca Lindell

Imaging description

Pleural lipomas are benign, rare, and asymptomatic tumors [1]. The pleural location and fat content of a pleural lipoma is not always identifiable on chest radiographs [1]. CT will show a well-defined, homogeneous, fat attenuation mass (HU less than −50) with obtuse margins along the pleura, which displaces adjacent pulmonary parenchyma [1, 2] [Figures 66.1–66.4]. Pleural lipomas are hyperintense on T1-weighted images and moderately intense on T2-weighted images on MRI [1].

Importance

A pleural lipoma is usually inconsequential but may present a diagnostic dilemma on radiographs and, rarely, CT as they must be distinguished from other causes of a nodule or mass.

Typical clinical scenario

Pleural lipomas are asymptomatic benign tumors usually incidentally imaged [1–3].

Differential diagnosis

Differential diagnoses would include other pleural tumors such as metastasis, fibrous tumor of the pleura, lymphoma, or mesothelioma, as well as parenchymal or chest wall tumors. CT can readily distinguish a pleural lipoma from these other entities. Rarely a pleural liposarcoma must be distinguished from a pleural lipoma on CT. Findings that suggest liposarcoma include a heterogeneous mix of fat and solid attenuation on CT or MRI [1, 2].

Teaching point

Pleural lipomas are rare, benign, and asymptomatic tumors usually incidentally imaged. Smooth margination, fat attenuation, and extrapulmonary location on CT chest or MRI can make a definitive diagnosis.

REFERENCES

1. Qureshi NR, Gleeson FV. Imaging of pleural disease. *Clin Chest Med* 2006; **27**: 193–213.
2. Muller NL. Imaging of the pleura. *Radiology* 1993; **186**: 297–309.
3. Gaerte SC, Meyer CA, Winer-Muram HT, Tarver RD, Conces DJ. Fat-containing lesions of the chest. *Radiographics* 2002; **22**: S61–S78.

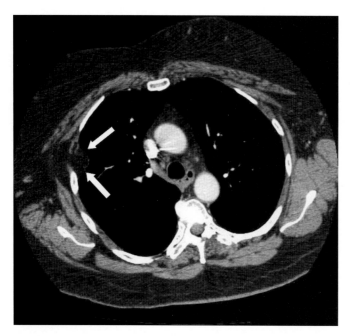

Figure 66.1 Axial contrast-enhanced CT chest image shows a fat attenuation nodule (arrows) arising from the pleura consistent with a pleural lipoma.

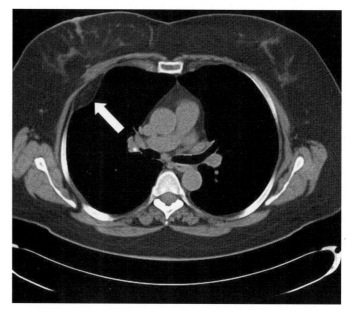

Figure 66.2 Axial image from a CT chest without contrast shows a pleural lipoma (arrow).

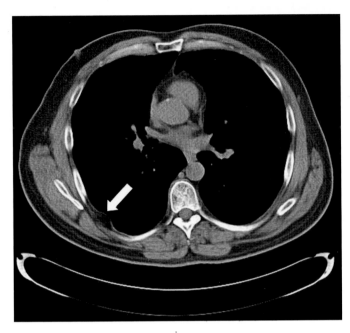

Figure 66.3 Noncontrast axial CT shows a small pleural lipoma (arrow).

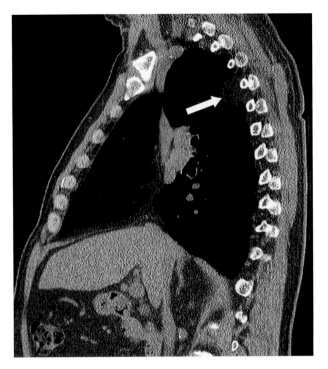

Figure 66.4 Sagittal reconstruction of a noncontrast CT chest shows a pleural lipoma (arrow) along the posterior upper right hemithorax, which was described as an indeterminate mass on chest radiograph.

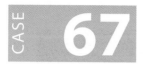
Prominent subpleural fat with chronic pleural disease

Thomas Hartman

Imaging

In the setting of a focal or diffuse pleural abnormality, the underlying subpleural fat can be thickened (Figures 67.1–67.3). This is likely due to hypertrophy secondary to chronic inflammation. As such, the presence of thickening of the subpleural fat is a strong indicator of chronic and, therefore, benign pleural disease (1–4). However, it should be stressed that thickened subpleural fat is not seen with every case of benign pleural disease and therefore the absence of thickening of the subpleural fat is not indicative of malignancy.

Importance

Recognition of thickened subpleural fat adjacent to a pleural abnormality is a strong predictor that the associated pleural abnormality is benign.

Typical clinical scenario

A pleural abnormality is detected on CT and raises the question of whether the pleural abnormality is benign or malignant.

Differential diagnosis

Although lipomas can present as focal accumulations of fat, they typically arise from the pleura and abut the lung.

Thickened subpleural fat is separated from the lung by the pleura and is therefore not typically confused with other entities.

Teaching point

While there are imaging findings of a pleural abnormality itself that can suggest a benign or malignant etiology, the presence of thickened subpleural fat adjacent to the pleural abnormality is a strong indicator that the pleural abnormality is benign.

REFERENCES

1. Metintas M, Ucgun I, Elbek O, et al. Computed tomography features in malignant pleural mesothelioma and other commonly seen pleural diseases. *Eur J Radiology* 2002; **41**: 1–9.
2. Leung AN, Muller NL, Miller RR. CT in differential diagnosis of diffuse pleural disease. *AJR Am J Roentgenol* 1990; **154**: 487–492.
3. Muller NL. Imaging of the pleura. *Radiology* 1993; **186**: 298–309.
4. Aberle DR, Balmes JR. Computed tomography of asbestos-related pulmonary parenchymal and pleural diseases. *Clin Chest Med* 1991; **12**: 115–131.

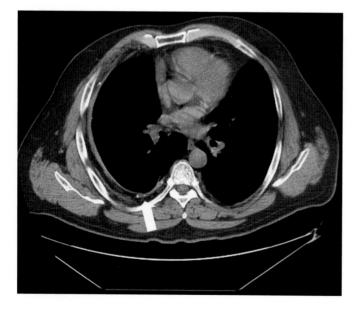

Figure 67.1 CT chest showing partially calcified pleural thickening on the right. There is hypertrophy of the subpleural fat on the right (arrow) indicating the pleural disease is likely benign.

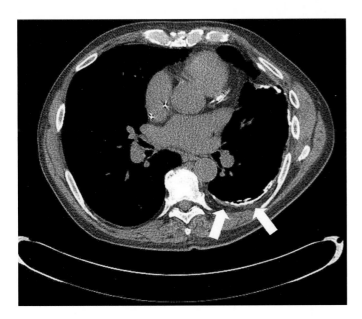

Figure 67.2 CT chest showing calcified pleural thickening on the left. There is hypertrophy of the subpleural fat on the left (arrows) indicating the pleural disease is likely benign.

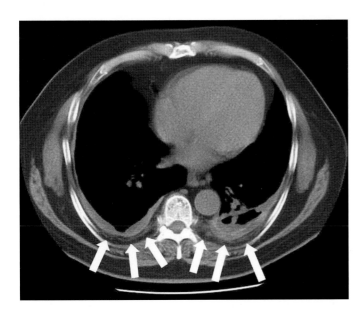

Figure 67.3 CT in a man with chronic pulmonary and pleural *Aspergillus* infection with recurrent bronchopleural fistulas. Axial image shows a small loculated left hydropneumothorax and bilateral complex pleural fluid and thickening with thickening of the adjacent subpleural fat (arrows).

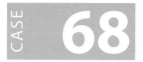

Benign fibrous tumor of the pleura (+/− pedicles)

Rebecca Lindell and Thomas Hartman

Imaging description

Benign fibrous tumors of the pleura are rare tumors of mesenchymal origin that are typically solitary and slow growing [1–3]. They may widely range in size and most often occur in the inferior hemithorax [1–3]. On radiographs as well as CT, the tumor may change location with time, patient position or respiration as 40% have a vascular pedicle that attaches it to the pleural surface and allows mobility within the pleural space [1–4]. On CT, smaller tumors are usually of homogeneous attenuation similar to muscle, with smooth, tapering margins and obtuse angles with the pleura (Figures 68.1 and 68.2) [1, 2, 5]. Larger tumors may be heterogeneous, are more often lobulated, and may form an acute angle to the pleural surface [1, 2, 5] (Figure 68.2). CT enhancement may occur and is often homogeneous in smaller tumors but may be heterogeneous in tumors with necrosis, myxoid degeneration, or hemorrhage [5]. Calcification occurs in less than 10% of cases. When present, it is usually punctate and occurs in the larger tumors [2]. Associated pleural effusions may occur [1, 2].

Importance

In patients with symptoms, confusion may exist with pleural malignancy. Removal of the tumor is usually curative.

Typical clinical scenario

The mean age at presentation is 50–60 years and there may be a slight female predominance [1, 2]. About half of patients with a benign fibrous tumor of the pleura are asymptomatic and the tumor is incidentally noted on radiographs or CT [5]. When present, symptoms may be due to localized effects or systemic effects. Symptoms relating to localized effect are more common in larger tumors [2, 5]. The most common symptoms are dyspnea, chest pain, cough, weight loss, and hypoglycemia. Less common symptoms include sweats, weakness, fatigue, clubbing, and upper respiratory infection and hypertrophic pulmonary osteoarthropathy [1, 5, 6].

Differential diagnosis

The differential of benign fibrous tumors of the pleura on CT includes other pleural nodules or masses such as metastasis, lymphoma, or mesothelioma. If the tumor abuts the mediastinum, mediastinal lesions must also be in the differential, such as neurogenic tumors or even extramedullary hematopoiesis. Movement of a pedunculated benign fibrous tumor on imaging suggests the correct diagnosis. Large tumors may still be difficult to differentiate from pulmonary masses on CT because of the acute angles they form with the pleural surface [3]. These tumors must also be distinguished from malignant fibrous tumors of the pleura. CT findings of malignant fibrous tumors include a diameter greater than 10 cm, necrosis, and ipsilateral pleural effusion [3].

Teaching point

Benign fibrous tumors of the pleura are rare, slow-growing tumors that vary in size. It typically appears as smooth or lobulated nodule or mass in the inferior hemithorax. The tumor may be pedunculated, which may allow it to change position with time, respiration, or patient position.

REFERENCES
1. Rosado-de-Christenson ML, Abbott GF, McAdams HP, Franks TJ, Galvin JR. From the archives of the AFIP: localized fibrous tumor of the pleura. *Radiographics* 2003; **23**(3): 759–783.
2. Qureshi NR, Gleeson FV. Imaging of pleural disease. *Clin Chest Med* 2006; **27**: 193–213.
3. Ferretti GR, Chiles C, Choplin RH, Coulomb M. Localized benign fibrous tumors of the pleura. *AJR Am J Roentgenol* 1997; **169**(3): 683–686.
4. Lee KS, Im J, Choe KO, Kim CJ, Lee BH. CT findings in benign fibrous mesothelioma of the pleura: pathologic correlation in nine patients. *AJR Am J Roentgenol* 1992; **158**: 983–986.
5. England DM, Hochholzer L, McCarthy MJ. Localized benign and malignant fibrous tumors of the pleura. A clinicopathologic review of 223 cases. *Am J Surg Pathol* 1989; **13**: 640–658.
6. Robinson LA. Solitary fibrous tumor of the pleura. *Cancer Control* 2006; **13**: 264–269.

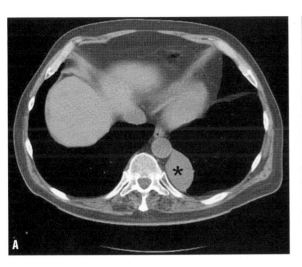 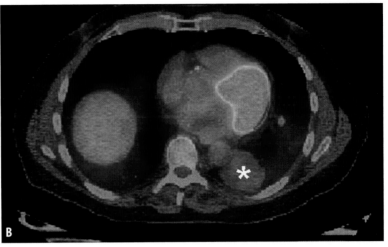

Figure 68.1 A. Noncontrast CT chest shows a homogeneous mass in the posterior left hemithorax (asterisk). The smooth, tapering margins with obtuse angles along the pleura help localize it as a pleural tumor. This was surgically removed and was a benign fibrous tumor of the pleura. **B.** PET/CT fusion scan shows that the mass (asterisk) has only minimal metabolic activity.

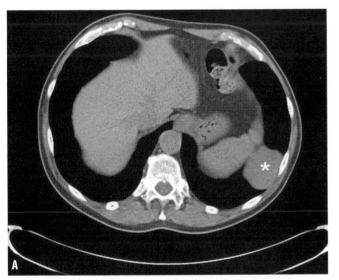 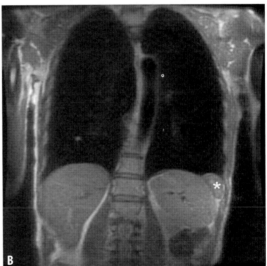

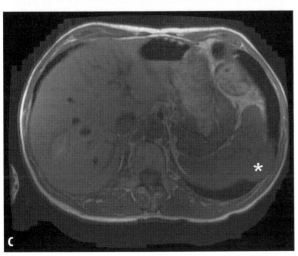

Figure 68.2 A. Axial image from a noncontrast CT chest shows an approximately 6.5 cm smoothly marginated homogeneous mass (asterisk) abutting the left hemidiaphragm forming acute angles with the pleura laterally. The mass was present but had grown 1 cm compared to a CT scan from 4 years prior. **B.** Coronal T2-weighted MRI shows the mass (asterisk) to be of intermediate to low signal intensity. Coronal images allow better determination of extrapulmonary location of the mass. **C.** Axial T1-weighted MRI shows the mass (asterisk) to be of low signal intensity.

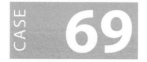

Talc pleurodesis

Rebecca Lindell

Imaging description

Talc pleurodesis is used to manage symptomatic benign and malignant pleural effusions, as well as recurrent pneumothoraces [1, 2]. Talc can be administered via chest tube or by insufflation during thoracoscopy [1]. It works by inciting an inflammatory reaction that results in adherence of the visceral and parietal pleura [2]. CT after talc pleurodesis typically shows high-attenuation areas along the pleura, more often linear than nodular, that are often most prominent in the posterior basal regions [2]. The high-attenuation material may also extend up to the apices, along the mediastinum, or within the fissures [Figures 69.1 and 69.2] [2]. The appearance of talc pleurodesis deposits on CT remains unchanged over time [2, 3]. Patients with residual pleural effusion may demonstrate high-attenuation talc along both the parietal and visceral surfaces around the pleural effusion on CT, giving a variant of the split pleura sign [2]. Talc pleurodesis deposits may show increased FDG uptake on PET, presumably due to secondary pleural inflammation [3, 4].

Importance

Correct identification of the CT appearance of talc pleurodesis is important not only for the sake of accuracy, but also because adhesions from a prior talc pleurodesis procedure may complicate or preclude thoracoscopy or lung transplantation [1]. In addition, it is important to not confuse imaging findings of talc pleurodesis with more serious diseases such as empyema or metastases [2–4].

Typical clinical scenario

Talc pleurodesis can be found in patients with a clinical history of recurrent pneumothoraces or benign or malignant pleural effusion. Surgical history is obviously very helpful in these patients.

Differential diagnosis

CT findings of talc pleurodesis may be confused with causes of pleural calcifications such as asbestos exposure, prior empyema, or prior trauma [1, 2]. Asbestos plaques typically are bilateral, while changes of talc pleurodesis occur only on the treated side [1, 2]. In addition, asbestos plaques tend to occur in the anterolateral and posteromedial aspects of the thorax [2]. Unlike talc pleurodesis changes, pleural calcifications caused by prior infection or trauma tend to be more extensive and coarse or plate-like [1, 2]. The talc pleurodesis variant of the split pleura sign (deposition of talc along the parietal and visceral pleural surfaces surrounding a pleural effusion) may mimic an empyema [2]. In such a case, surgical history, clinical symptoms, and the high attenuation of the talc would help distinguish these entities. Talc deposits may be FDG positive on PET and could be confused with pleural metastases [3, 4]. However, correlation between PET and CT imaging as well as clinical history is usually sufficient to differentiate these cases.

Teaching point

Prior talc pleurodesis may be demonstrated on CT as linear and/or nodular high-attenuation areas along the pleural surface of the treated hemithorax. It is usually most prominent in the dependent basal regions of the hemithorax but may extend anywhere along the pleura. It may be PET positive. Knowledge of its imaging appearance and clinical history can help distinguish it from causes of pleural calcification or more serious disease entities.

REFERENCES

1. Murray JG, Patz EF Jr, Erasmus JJ, Gilkeson RC. CT appearance of the pleural space after talc pleurodesis. *AJR Am J Roentgenol* 1997; **169**: 89–91.

2. Narayanaswamy S, Kamath S, Williams M. CT appearances of talc pleurodesis. *Clin Radiol* 2007; **62**(3): 233–237.

3. Kwek BH, Aquino SL, Fischman AJ. Fluorodeoxyglucose positron emission tomography and CT after talc pleurodesis. *Chest* 2004; **125**(6): 2356–2360.

4. Murray JG, Erasmus JJ, Bahtiarian EA, Goodman PC. Talc pleurodesis simulating pleural metastases on 18F-fluorodeoxyglucose positron emission tomography. *AJR Am J Roentgenol* 1997; **168**: 359–360.

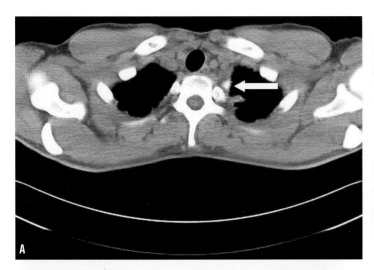

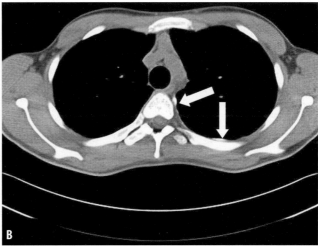

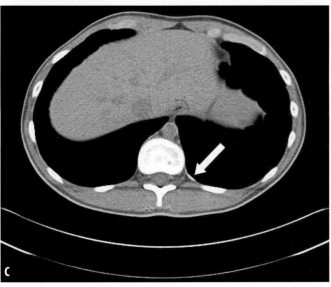

Figures 69.1 A.–C. Axial images from a noncontrast CT chest in a man with a history of recurrent spontaneous pneumothoraces, who had been treated with talc pleurodesis. There is high-attenuation material (arrows) along the pleural surface of the medial and posterior upper left hemithorax and in the posteromedial left base, compatible with prior talc pleurodesis.

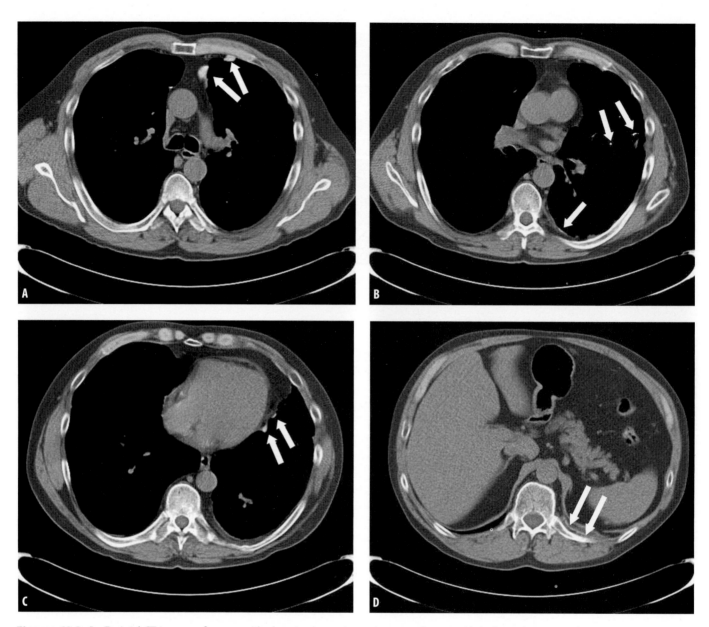

Figures 69.2 A.–D. Axial CT images of a man with chronic obstructive pulmonary disease with bullous changes and recurrent pneumothoraces. There are nodular and linear areas of high attenuation material (arrows) along the pleural surface on the left, including along the inferior aspect of the left major fissure, compatible with prior talc pleurodesis.

Morgagni hernia

Rebecca Lindell

Imaging description

Morgagni hernia is an uncommon hernia resulting from a defect in the diaphragm's attachments to the sternum and costal cartilages with herniation of abdominal content into the anterior thorax [1, 2]. It more commonly occurs on the right due to the protective barrier effect of the heart on the left [1, 2]. On CT, the Morgagni foraminal defect is demonstrated by the lack of right and left diaphragmatic muscle fibers joining together to insert on the xiphoid [3] (Figure 70.1).

The hernia most commonly contains omentum but may contain colon, stomach, liver, or small intestine [1, 2] (Figures 70.2–70.4).

Importance

Morgagni hernias comprise 2–3% of all diaphragmatic hernias [1]. They are usually inconsequential, but may occasionally cause nonspecific symptoms and need repair (Figures 70.3 and 70.4). They need to be distinguished from other causes of a cardiophrenic angle mass.

Typical clinical scenario

Morgagni hernias typically occur in adults and may be associated with obesity, trauma, or other causes of increased intra-abdominal pressure [2]. Most are asymptomatic and are incidentally found on imaging. When symptomatic, the symptoms are nonspecific and relate to one or more organ systems involved in the hernia such as gastrointestinal, respiratory, or cardiac [1].

Differential diagnosis

A Morgagni hernia is usually easy to distinguish from two of the other causes of cardiophrenic angle masses such as a pericardial cyst or solid tumor/adenopathy [4]. It may be slightly more difficult to distinguish from a prominent fat pad in the cardiophrenic angle, but careful attenuation to the presence or absence of the diaphragmatic muscle fibers insertion on the xiphoid will establish the diagnosis. Presence of abdominal contents within the mass will also allow differentiation of a Morgagni hernia [2] from a prominent fat pad. Occasionally, fat or bowel loops may project anterior to the heart on CT with an intact diaphragm as a normal variant. In these cases, it again will be important to identify the right and left diaphragmatic muscle fibers joining together to insert on the xiphoid above this fat or bowel loop in order to exclude a hernia [3].

Teaching point

Morgagni hernias are a cause of a cardiophrenic angle mass and typically occur on the right side. They are usually incidental but may occasionally cause nonspecific symptoms relating to the affected organ systems. Absence of the diaphragmatic muscle insertions on the xiphoid on CT imaging will allow diagnosis.

REFERENCES

1. LaRosa DV Jr, Esham RH, Morgan SL, Wing SW. Diaphragmatic hernia of Morgagni. *South Med J* 1999; **92**: 409–411.
2. Tarver RD, Conces DJ Jr, Cory DA, Vix VA. Imaging of the diaphragm and its disorders. *J Thorac Imaging* 1989; **4**(1): 1–18.
3. Gale ME. Anterior diaphragm: variations in the CT appearance. *Radiology* 1986; **161**: 635–639.
4. Gaerte SC, Meyer CA, Winer-Muram HT, Tarver RD, Conces, DJ. Fat-containing lesions of the chest. *Radiographics* 2002; **22**: S61–S78.

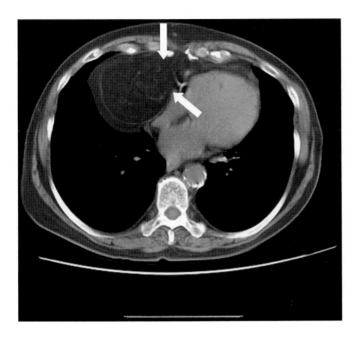

Figure 70.1 Axial image from a CT chest shows a mass composed of fat protruding from the abdomen, compatible with a Morgagni hernia. Arrows point to the diaphragmatic defect.

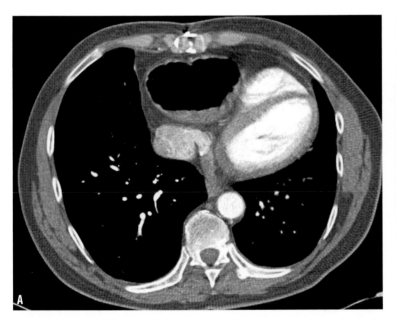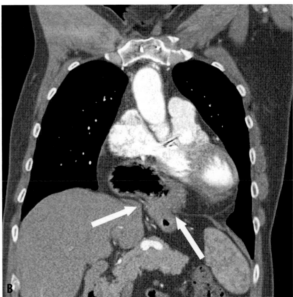

Figure 70.2 A. Axial image from a CT chest with intravenous contrast shows the stomach in the lower anterior mediastinum causing mass effect on the heart. **B.** Coronal image from the same CT chest as Figure 70.2A better depicts the diaphragmatic defect (arrows) with the stomach herniating into the chest.

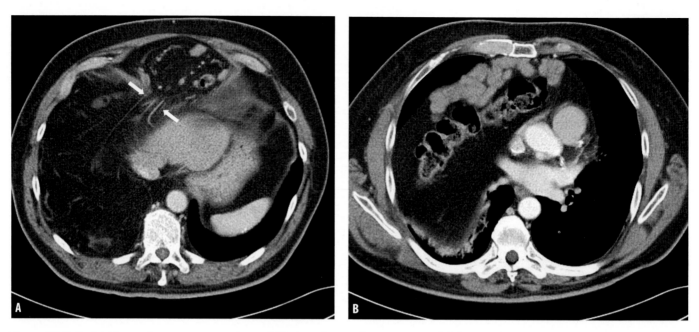

Figure 70.3 A. Axial image from a contrast-enhanced CT chest shows a large amount of abdominal fat and vessels herniating into the right hemithorax via a Morgagni hernia defect. Note the absence of convergence of the diaphragmatic muscles into the xiphoid (arrows). **B.** Axial image from the same CT as Figure 70.3A shows that the hernia contains portions of the colon and small bowel.

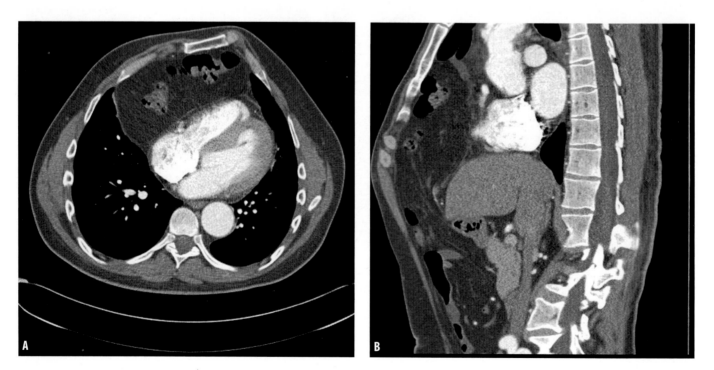

Figure 70.4 A. Axial image from a CT chest shows the transverse colon, vessels, and a large amount of abdominal fat herniating into the anterior thorax via a Morgagni hernia defect. **B.** Sagittal image from the same CT as 70.4A again shows the transverse colon, vessels, and a large amount of abdominal fat herniating into the anterior thorax via a Morgagni hernia defect.

Bochdalek hernia

Rebecca Lindell

Imaging description

A Bochdalek hernia is a defect of the posterior hemidiaphragm with protrusion of abdominal content, usually fat, into the thorax [1]. It may occur on either side, but is more common on the left side due to a protective barrier effect of the liver [1, 2]. CT typically demonstrates the diaphragmatic defect with abdominal fat or omentum protruding through the defect [1–4] (Figure 71.1). Less commonly, retroperitoneal or intra-peritoneal organs may herniate through the defect [3] (Figures 71.2 and 71.3). The kidney is the most common organ to herniate through the defect, followed by the spleen [3].

Importance

Bochdalek hernias are present in approximately 6% of adults, with incidence increasing with age [2]. The vast majority of Bochdalek hernias occurring in adults are inconsequential [1, 2]. Rarely, incarceration of hernia content may occur [3]. Lack of familiarity with the typical imaging appearance of a Bochdalek hernia may lead to unnecessary work up as it may be mistaken for an indeterminate mass or diaphragmatic injury.

Typical clinical scenario

Bochdalek hernias are typically an incidental finding on chest radiograph or CT [4]. They may be bilateral or unilateral but typically occur on the left [1, 4].

Differential diagnosis

The imaging findings on CT are usually diagnostic. However, in the setting of trauma, it may be difficult to distinguish a diaphragmatic hernia from a rupture. Sagittal and/or coronal reconstructions may be helpful [1].

Teaching point

Bochdalek hernias are typically an asymptomatic, incidental finding on CT and should not be mistaken for an indeterminate mass.

REFERENCES

1. Gaerte SC, Meyer CA, Winer-Muram HT, et al. Fat-containing lesions of the chest. *Radiographics* 2002; **22**: S61–S78.
2. Gale ME. Bochdalek hernia: prevalence and CT characteristics. *Radiology* 1985; **156**: 449–452.
3. Mullins ME, Stein J, Saini SS, Mueller PR. Prevalence of incidental Bochdalek's hernia in a large adult population. *AJR Am J Roentgenol* 2001; **177**: 363–366.
4. Tarver RD, Conces DJ Jr, Cory DA, Vix VA. Imaging of the diaphragm and its disorders. *J Thorac Imaging* 1989; **4**(1): 1–18.

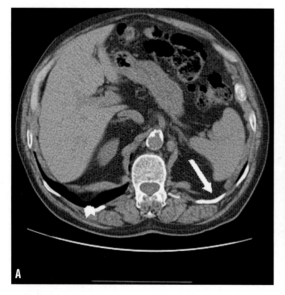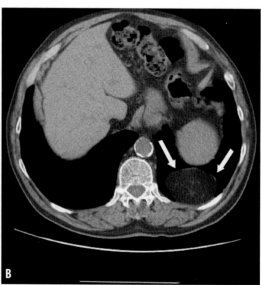

Figure 71.1 A. CT chest without intravenous contrast reveals a defect in the posterior left hemidiaphragm (arrow) with abdominal fat protruding through the defect, compatible with a Bochdalek hernia. There was also a Bochdalek hernia on the right (arrowhead), but the diaphragmatic defect was on a lower image (not shown). **B.** Axial CT image from the same study shows that a large amount of fat on the left (arrows) has herniated from the abdomen.

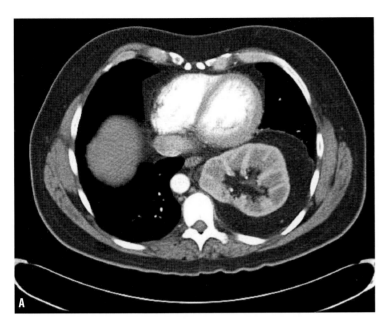
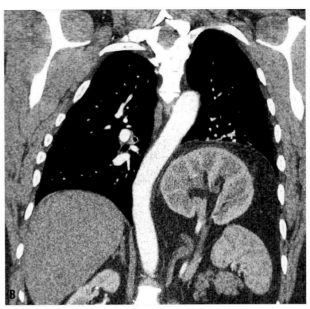

Figure 71.2 **A.** Axial contrast-enhanced CT image of the chest shows a Bochdalek hernia on the left containing the left kidney. **B.** Coronal reconstruction from the CT chest shows the discontinuity of the left hemidiaphragm with herniation of the kidney and its vascular pedicle through the defect as well as a portion of the spleen.

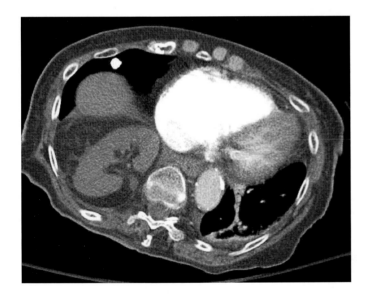

Figure 71.3 Axial contrast-enhanced CT chest shows a right Bochdalek hernia containing the right kidney.

Imaging description

The cysterna chyli is a lymphatic sac formed by the confluence of lumbar lymphatic ducts. It is the origin (caudal-most aspect) of the thoracic duct [1]. It is in the right retrocrural space usually at the T11–L2 level [1]. The confluence of the lumbar lymphatic channels occasionally (1.7%) will form a distinct tubular structure on CT [2] and can appear as a round or elliptical opacity 4–9 mm (average 7 mm) in size [2]. On CT it has attenuation similar to that of water [1, 2] (Figure 72.1). On MRI it has signal intensity similar to that of bile or cerebrospinal fluid [3] and can have many different shapes including round, oval, sausage-shaped, or a focal plexus [3].

Importance

A prominent cysterna chyli can simulate a low-attenuation enlarged lymph node or focal retrocrural fluid collection.

Typical clinical scenario

Focal fluid attenuation is incidentally seen on CT or MRI to the right of the aorta in the right retrocrural space adjacent to the azygos and hemiazygos veins.

Differential diagnosis

Low-attenuation lymph node or focal fluid collection. However, its fluid attenuation, tubular shape, and location are usually diagnostic.

Teaching point

Prominent cysterna chyli is dilatation of the confluence of abdominal lymphatics that forms the start of the thoracic duct at the T11–L2 level. Its fluid attenuation and location in the right retrocrural space should be diagnostic.

REFERENCES

1. Gollub MJ, Castellino RA. The cisterna chyli: a potential mimic of retrocrural lymphadenopathy on CT scans. *Radiology* 1996; **199**(2): 477–480.
2. Smith TR, Grigoropoulos J. The cisterna chyli: incidence and characteristics on CT. *Clin Imaging* 2002; **26**(1): 18–22.
3. Pinto PS, Sirlin CB, Andrade-Barreto OA, et al. Cisterna chyli at routine abdominal MR imaging: a normal anatomic structure in the retrocrural space. *Radiographics* 2004; **24**(3): 809–817.

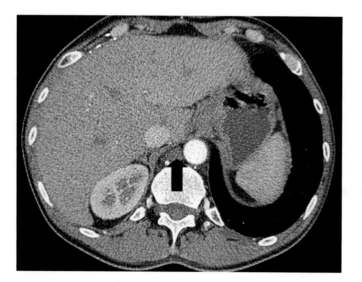

Figure 72.1 Contrast-enhanced CT chest shows a rounded fluid attenuation structure (arrow) located between the azygos vein and aorta in the right retrocrural space at the T12 level.

Diffuse pulmonary lymphangiomatosis

John Hildebrandt

Imaging description

Diffuse pulmonary lymphangiomatosis (DPL) is a disease of uncertain etiology that results in an increase in number and dilatation of the lymphatic channels. CT findings consist of smooth thickening of the interlobular septa and bronchovascular interstitium bilaterally (Figure 73.1A), [1]. Chylous pleural effusions and pleural thickening are common (Figure 73.1A) [1]. Mediastinal adenopathy and increased attenuation of mediastinal fat may also be present (Figure 73.1B), [1].

Importance

DPL accounts for approximately 5% of all chronic interstitial lung disease, presents in the pediatric to young adult population, and causes a restrictive and/or obstructive lung disease [2, 3].

Typical clinical scenario

DPL generally presents as asthma, wheezing, or dyspnea in the pediatric population. It occurs with equal frequency in males and females. Pulmonary function test can show abnormalities of restriction, obstruction, or both.

Differential diagnosis

DPL can have a similar appearance to interstitial edema, pulmonary veno-occlusive disease (PVOD), or lymphangitic carcinomatosis. Edema typically has associated cardiomegaly and pulmonary venous enlargement which are absent in DPL.

PVOD typically also has areas of ground-glass attenuation and enlargement of the central pulmonary arteries which are absent in DPL. Lymphangitic carcinomatosis typically has nodular thickening of the interlobular septa and may be unilateral instead of bilateral. The combination of smooth interlobular septal thickening, increased attenuation of mediastinal fat and/or adenopathy, and associated pleural thickening or effusion in the absence of the other findings listed above usually allows differentiation of DPL from the other diseases.

> ## Teaching point
>
> DPL is a chronic interstitial lung disease of children caused by dilatation and increase in number of lymphatic channels of the lung. It causes smooth diffuse interlobular septal thickening commonly accompanied by pleural effusions which are often chylous effusions.

REFERENCES

1. Swenson SJ, Hartman TE, Mayo JR, et al. Diffuse pulmonary lymphangiomatosis: CT findings. *J Comput Assist Tomogr* 1995; **19**(3): 348–352.
2. Fall LL, Mullen AL, Brugman SM, et al. Clinical spectrum of chronic interstitial lung disease in children. *J Pediatr* 1992; **121**(6): 867–872.
3. Tazelaar HD, Kerr D, Yousem SA, et al. Diffuse pulmonary lymphangiomatosis. *Hum Pathol* 1993; **24**(12): 1313–1322.

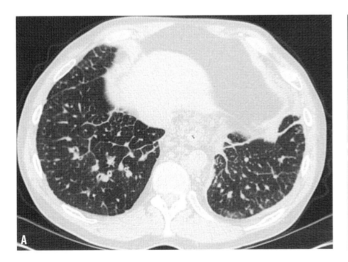
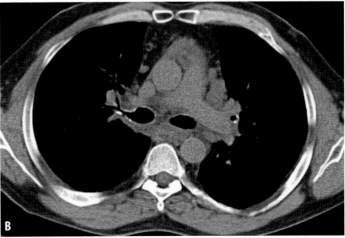

Figure 73.1 **A.** Axial CT in patient with biopsy-proven diffuse pulmonary lymphangiomatosis. High-resolution CT shows smooth interlobular septa, bronchovascular thickening, and mosaic attenuation consistent with air trapping. Patient had severe obstruction on pulmonary function testing. Left pleural thickening is also present. **B.** CT shows mediastinal adenopathy and increased attenuation of mediastinal fat.

Lymphangitic carcinomatosis

John Hildebrandt

Imaging description

Lymphangitic carcinomatosis typically affects the central (perihilar) and peripheral lymphatic system of the lung [1]. Centrally there is thickening along the arteries and bronchi (i.e., peribronchovascular interstitium) (Figure 74.1). Peripherally there is thickening of the interlobular septa. This smooth thickening can be a result of either tumor or edema due to lymphatic obstruction. Less common, but more specific is nodular or beaded thickening of these spaces [1, 2] (Figure 74.2). On CT, hilar or mediastinal lymph node enlargement is present in approximately 40% of cases and pleural effusion in 30% [3]. Lung involvement may be bilateral (Figure 74.2), but is found to be asymmetrical (Figure 74.3) or unilateral in approximately 50% [3]. Unilateral involvement is most often caused by bronchogenic carcinoma [3] (Figure 74.1). Additional findings may include hematogenous metastatic disease (Figure 74.3) or identification of the primary tumor.

Importance

Lymphangitic carcinomatosis is a common presentation of metastatic disease in the chest. The presentation of nodular interlobular septal thickening can be diagnostic.

Typical clinical scenario

Progressive dyspnea and cough usually in patients with a known malignancy. Malignancies that commonly present with lymphangitic carcinomatosis include breast, renal, stomach, pancreas, prostate, and lung.

Differential diagnosis

The primary differential consideration is pulmonary edema. Other potential diagnoses include sarcoidosis and diffuse pulmonary lymphangiomatosis. However, if there is nodular thickening the diagnosis of lymphangitic carcinomatosis is likely.

Teaching point

Lymphangitic carcinomatosis is a common mode of spread of malignancy in the lung. It typically presents as interlobular septal and peribronchovascular interstitial thickening. When the interlobular septal thickening is nodular it is highly suggestive of the diagnosis.

REFERENCES

1. Johkoh T, Ikezoe J, Tomiyama N, et al. CT findings in lymphangitic carcinomatosis of the lung: correlation with histologic findings and pulmonary function tests. *AJR Am J Roentgenol* 1992; **158**: 1217–1222.

2. Ren H, Hruban RH, Kuhlman JE, et al. Computed tomography of inflation-fixed lungs: the beaded septum sign of pulmonary metastases. *J Comput Assist Tomogr* 1989; **13**(3): 411–416.

3. Munk PL, Muller NL, Miller RR, Ostrow DN. Pulmonary lymphangitic carcinomatosis: CT and pathologic findings. *Radiology* 1988; **166**(3): 705–709.

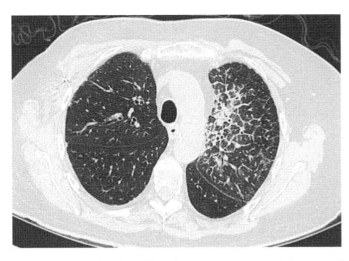

Figure 74.1 CT of unilateral lymphangitic carcinomatosis in a case of lung cancer. Interlobular septal thickening in the left lung, most prominent in the left perihilar region.

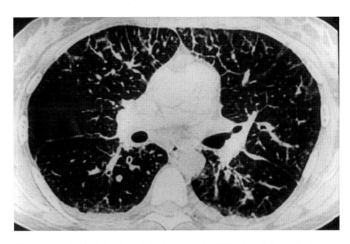

Figure 74.2 Nodular interlobular septal thickening bilaterally in a case of lymphangitic carcinomatosis secondary to vaginal adenocarcinoma.

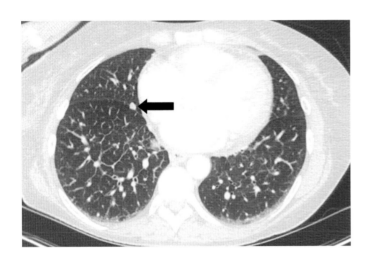

Figure 74.3 CT in a woman with renal cell carcinoma demonstrates smooth thickening of the interlobular septa bilaterally, greater on the right. There is also a hematogenous metastatic nodule in the right middle lobe posteriorly (arrow).

Pulmonary nodule misregistration on PET/CT

Patrick Peller

Imaging description

The CT in an integrated PET/CT scanner is optimized for PET imaging. The CT is converted to provide attenuation correction and to lend structural data to the fused PET/CT image. Accurate co-registration between the CT and PET images is optimal for both attenuation correction and fusion. The CT images are generally acquired at mid-inspiration and PET images are acquired during quiet respiration. Careful patient coaching and cooperation is required to prevent a mismatch between the two datasets. Pulmonary nodules, particularly in the lung bases, have modest motion even with quiet breathing. The net result is that "hot spot" on the PET image does not match the lung nodule on the CT image. Review of the CT slices above and below the hot focus allows confident identification of this artifact (Figure 75.1). The frequency of misregistration is lessened when PET/CT is performed on scanners with six or more rows of CT detectors [1, 2].

Importance

Incorrect localization of a pulmonary FDG "hot spot" in the lungs could have several adverse consequences. At a minimum, the error is confusing, since there will be no anatomic correlate for the foci of increased FDG uptake in the lungs on CT. Worse, a patient may be incorrectly assumed to have low FDG uptake in the pulmonary nodule so that the nodule is not reported as having high malignant potential.

Typical clinical scenario

This artifactual misregistration typically occurs when a patient has a pulmonary nodule in the lower third of the lung fields or is breathing deeply during the CT exam. The FDG uptake in the lung nodule is often "smeared" across multiple axial slices and does not match with the CT nodule location. The misregistration and smearing may produce a SUV measurement that is artifactually low.

Differential diagnosis

Review of the PET slices above and below the CT lung nodule allows confident identification of this artifact. The hot clot artifact can appear similar, but there is no pulmonary nodule on CT.

> ## Teaching point
>
> Pulmonary nodules with no corresponding FDG uptake on PET images of a PET/CT study should prompt careful review of the adjacent axial images, since the finding may represent misregistration.

REFERENCES

1. Bockisch A, Beyer T, Antoch G, et al. Positron emission tomography/computed tomography–imaging protocols, artifacts and pitfalls. *Mol Imaging Biol* 2004; **6**(4): 188–199.

2. Beyer T, Rosenbaum S, Veit P, et al. Respiration artifacts in whole-body (18)F-FDG PET/CT studies with combined PET/CT tomographs employing spiral CT technology with 1 to 16 detector rows. *Eur J Nucl Med Mol Imaging* 2005; **32**(12): 1429–1439.

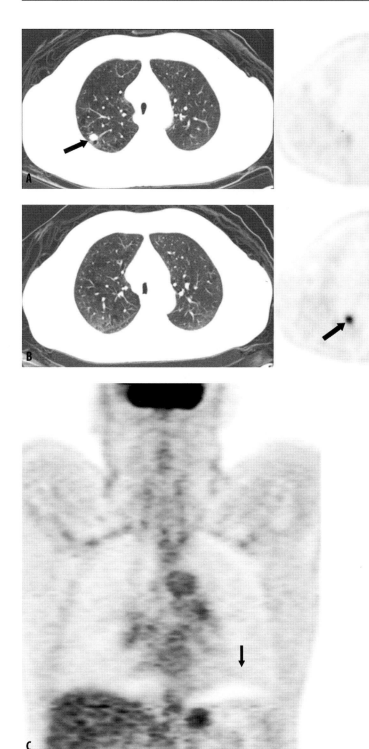

Figure 75.1 This 67-year-old male presents for evaluation of a right lung pulmonary nodule. **A.** Corresponding axial CT and PET images show 1.2 cm by 1.0 cm right upper lung nodule (arrow) with minor FDG uptake. **B.** Corresponding axial CT and PET images three axial slices below Figure 75.1A demonstrate intense FDG uptake (arrow) and no lung nodule on CT. **C.** Attenuation corrected coronal FDG-PET image shows the degree of misregistration of the lungs in this patient. The white curvilinear areas near the diaphragm (arrow) and periphery of the lungs are the result of deep inspiration during CT scanning. This "cold" artifact should alert the interpreter that misregistration in the lungs and upper abdomen are possible.

Hot clot artifact

Patrick Peller

Imaging description

Some nuclear radiopharmaceuticals are notoriously sticky and will produce agglutination of red blood cells (RBCs) inadvertently drawn back into the syringe prior to tracer administration. FDG can glue a few RBCs together, which when administered intravenously, will lodge temporally in a small pulmonary artery. The clot formed at injection is usually small, short lived, and will have intense activity [1].

Importance

Incorrect interpretation of a hot lung focus could have severe adverse consequences. At a minimum, the hot clot is confusing, since there is no underlying pulmonary nodule on CT lung windows (Figure 76.1). Worse, the patient may be incorrectly interpreted to have a pulmonary metastasis, leading to incorrect staging and treatment.

Typical clinical scenario

This occurs when FDG is administered with a straight stick and a small amount of blood is drawn back into the syringe to insure satisfactory venous access. The FDG mixes with a small number of RBCs, which stick together and wedge within the pulmonary arterial system. The clot has intense activity since concentrated FDG binds the RBCs.

Differential diagnosis

The hot clot has a similar pattern as a pulmonary metastasis. Review of the CT slices above and below this hot focus allows confident identification of this artifact.

Teaching point

An apparent intensely FDG-avid pulmonary metastasis present only on the PET portion of the PET/CT study should prompt careful review of the CT lung windows for corresponding nodular density.

REFERENCE
1. Karantanis D, Subramaniam RM, Mullan BP, Peller PJ, Wiseman GA. Focal F-18 fluoro-deoxy-glucose accumulation in the lung parenchyma in the absence of CT abnormality in PET/CT. *J Comput Assist Tomogr* 2007; **31**(5): 800–805.

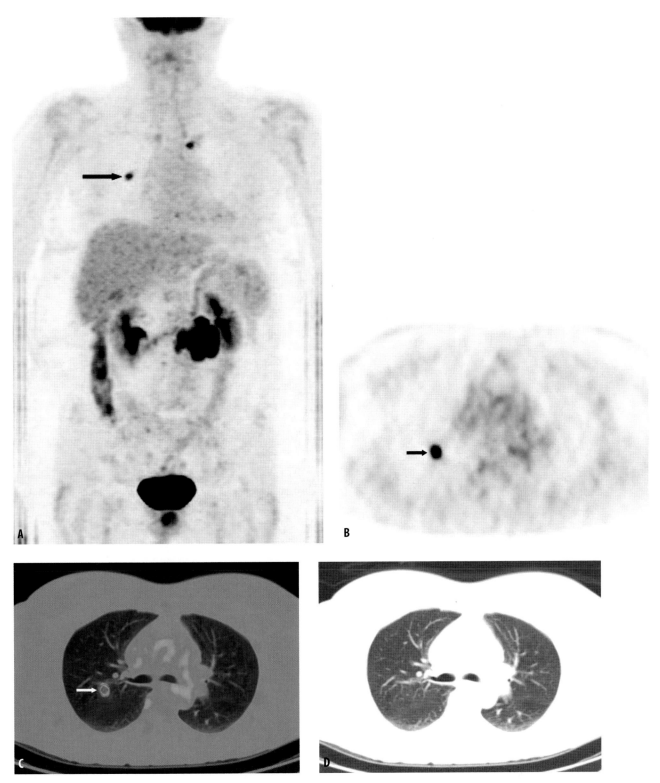

Figure 76.1 This 58-year-old male presents for restaging rectal cancer. **A.** Maximum intensity projection PET image demonstrates two intense foci of activity within the lungs, suggestive of metastases. **B.** Axial PET image demonstrates an intense focus adjacent to the right hilum (arrow). **C.** Fused axial PET/CT image demonstrates an intense focus of uptake in the adjacent right lung (arrow) suggestive of a metastasis. **D.** Corresponding axial CT image shows no right lung nodule at the site of FDG uptake. **E.** The axial CT images, above (left image) and below (right image) the hot PET focus, show no lung nodule and confirm the hot clot artifact.

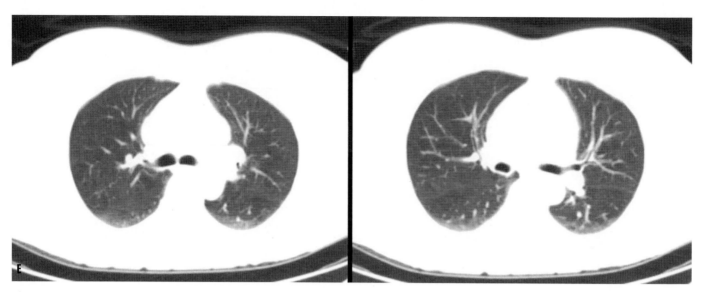

Figure 76.1 (cont.)

Brown fat on PET/CT

Patrick Peller

Imaging description

Brown adipose tissue is extremely important in regulating energy expenditure and maintaining normal body temperature in newborn infants. The absolute amount and percentage of brown fat versus white fat decreases with age. In the past, brown fat was not thought to play a role in adult temperature control. PET/CT scanning demonstrates the presence of brown fat activation in adults by intense FDG uptake (Figure 77.1). Colder temperatures and anxiety enhance FDG uptake. On PET/CT, FDG uptake in brown fat is predominantly located in the neck, supraclavicular and paravertebral areas, and is inversely related to body mass index (BMI) and percent body fat. Children and adolescents may have FDG uptake in brown fat in the upper abdomen and adjacent to the diaphragm [1–3].

Importance

The intense irregular FDG accumulation produced by brown fat activation can mimic nodal disease, potentially leading to unnecessary workup and treatment if misinterpreted. Alternatively, brown fat activation can obscure small or subtle foci of recurrent disease.

Typical clinical scenario

Patients under the age of 35 and BMI of less than 25 kg/m^2 during the colder months will present with fat activation on PET/CT scan. Even increasing the temperature of the uptake room to 75 °F and using prewarmed blankets at 160 °F may not prevent brown fat activation, especially in thin teens.

Differential diagnosis

Brown fat activation produces FDG uptake on PET images encompassing large areas of adipose tissue without underlying lymph nodes or masses on corresponding CT images. Nodal disease of lymphoma or metastatic cancer can produce a similar pattern of activity on PET/CT. If necessary, repeating the study with Valium pretreatment will usually ablate FDG accumulation in the adipose tissue, allowing differentiation of brown fat activation from malignancy [4].

Teaching point

Symmetric, moderate to intense multifocal FDG uptake in the adipose tissue of the neck and shoulders in a young patient is commonly due to brown fat activation.

REFERENCES

1. Paidisetty S, Blodgett TM. Brown fat: atypical locations and appearances encountered in PET/CT. *AJR Am J Roentgenol* 2009; **193**(2): 359–366.
2. Saito M, Okamatsu-Ogura Y, Matsushita M, et al. High incidence of metabolically active brown adipose tissue in healthy adult humans: effects of cold exposure and adiposity. *Diabetes* 2009; **58**(7): 1526–1531.
3. Cypess AM, Lehman S, Williams G, et al. Identification and importance of brown adipose tissue in adult humans. *N Engl J Med* 2009; **360**(15): 1509–1517.
4. Sturkenboom MG, Hoekstra OS, Postema EJ, et al. A randomised controlled trial assessing the effect of oral diazepam on 18F-FDG uptake in the neck and upper chest region. *Mol Imaging Biol* 2009; **11**(5): 364–368.

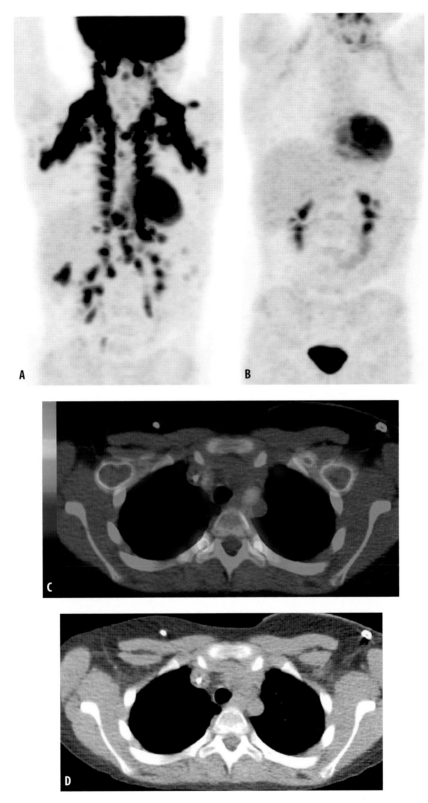

Figure 77.1 This 8-year-old male presents for evaluation following treatment for Burkitt's lymphoma. **A.** Maximum intensity projection (MIP) PET image demonstrates intense increased activity symmetrically in the neck, shoulders, back, and upper abdomen, typical of brown fat activation. **B.** Repeat MIP PET image the next day, following Valium pretreatment before bed and the morning of the scanning, shows marked decrease in the brown fat activation. **C.** Fused axial PET/CT image demonstrates intense activity within the axillae and paravertebral regions bilaterally. **D.** Corresponding axial CT image shows no nodal disease within the axillae.

78 Pulmonary Langerhans cell histiocytosis on PET/CT

Patrick Peller

Imaging description

Pulmonary Langerhans cell histiocytosis (PLCH) is a rare interstitial lung disease that primarily affects young adult smokers. PLCH begins as densely cellular, peribronchiolar nodules and has a characteristic predilection for the upper lungs. Treatment is cessation of smoking and corticosteroids in selected patients. In PLCH, CT classically shows a combination of nodules and cysts in the mid and upper lungs with sparing of the lung bases. PET scans show irregular, increased pulmonary activity corresponding to the nodular disease on CT (Figure 78.1). PLCH patients with a dominant cystic pattern and fewer nodules demonstrate less pulmonary FDG uptake [1–3].

Importance

The presenting symptoms of PLCH are very nonspecific, but the CT imaging findings are usually diagnostic. The presence of significant FDG uptake corresponds to a considerable inflammatory component to the disease and provides support for treatment with corticosteroids in addition to smoking cessation.

Typical clinical scenario

A smoker in their second or third decade of life presents with a persistent cough or dyspnea out of proportion to the findings on chest radiograph. High-resolution CT shows combination of multiple nodules and cysts with an upper lung predominance that spares the bases.

Differential diagnosis

In a young smoker, the combination of multiple cysts and nodules with sparing of the lung bases on CT is characteristic of PLCH. Nodular lung diseases that can spare the bases include: sarcoidosis, granulomatous infection, and silicosis. The upper lung predominance with basilar sparing would be atypical for metastatic disease. In cases with cystic disease only, the main differential is lymphangioleiomyomatosis (LAM). However, the diffuse distribution of the cysts in LAM allows differentiation from PLCH.

Teaching point

In young smokers, moderate diffuse FDG uptake in nodular disease involving the mid and upper lungs with sparing of the bases may be due to PLCH. Review of the CT images should allow a confident diagnosis of PLCH to be made.

REFERENCES

1. Vassallo R, Ryu JH, Colby TV, Hartman T, Limper AH. Pulmonary Langerhans'-cell histiocytosis. *N Engl J Med* 2000; **342**(26): 1969–1978.
2. Abbott GF, Rosado-de-Christenson ML, Franks TJ, Frazier AA, Galvin JR. From the archives of the AFIP: pulmonary Langerhans cell histiocytosis. *Radiographics* 2004; **24**(3): 821–841.
3. Krajicek BJ, Ryu JH, Hartman TE, Lowe VJ, Vassallo R. Abnormal fluorodeoxyglucose PET in pulmonary Langerhans cell histiocytosis. *Chest* 2009; **135**(6): 1542–1549.

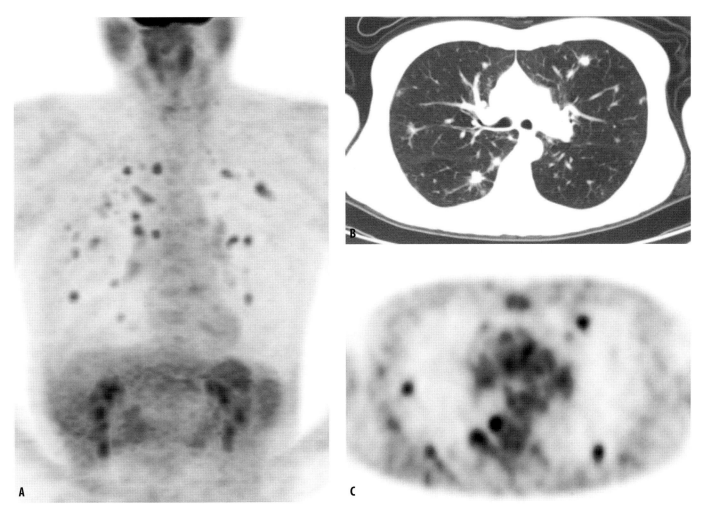

Figure 78.1 This 45-year-old male presents for evaluation of persistent shortness of breath. **A.** Maximum intensity projection PET image demonstrates numerous foci of increased activity within the lungs, especially the upper and mid lungs. **B.** Axial CT image demonstrates numerous nodules with minimal interstitial thickening in both lungs. **C.** Corresponding axial PET image shows intense increased activity within the nodules, typical of PLCH. The intense FDG uptake suggests that this patient is in the earlier stages of the disease process.

Talc pleurodesis on PET/CT

Patrick Peller

Imaging description

Talc pleurodesis is performed to obliterate the pleural space to prevent recurrent pleural effusion or spontaneous pneumothorax. All pleural fluid present is drained and talc is insufflated at thoracoscopy or instilled as a slurry by chest tube. Talc is a chemical irritant causing an intense inflammatory response. The leukocytes in this inflammatory response accumulate FDG avidly, outlining the talc-treated pleural. After months, the inflammation often becomes irregular along the pleural surface. This activity on PET lasts for years and possibly over a decade. The intense pleural activity mimics that seen in mesothelioma and pleural metastasis (Figure 79.1). The increased attenuation of talc can best be seen in the pleural reflections on CT [1, 2].

Importance

Incorrect interpretation of increased FDG accumulation along the pleura due to talc pleurodesis could have significant adverse consequences. The intense pleural uptake of FDG on PET/CT secondary to talc pleurodesis can be misinterpreted as recurrent or metastatic malignancy. The pleural activity from talc can obscure the evaluation of pleural disease and mesothelioma [3].

Typical clinical scenario

A patient with a known malignancy presents for follow-up months or years after initial diagnosis and treatment. The patient will often have no symptoms referable to the chest wall at the site of FDG accumulation. Minimal to no effusion or pleural thickening may be present. Since the pleural uptake from talc pleurodesis can persist for years the referring physician and the patient may not provide this crucial piece of history.

Differential diagnosis

The findings in talc pleurodesis are very similar to mesothelioma and pleural metastasis. In patients with mesothelioma, talc pleurodesis to treat recurrent pleural effusions limits future PET/CT evaluation since the activity of the tumor and the talc-induced inflammation will be similar. Careful review of the PET/CT images in the pleural reflections adjacent to the diaphragm is important to allow confident identification of flocculated talc at this site.

> ### Teaching point
>
> Apparent pleural metastases seen on PET/CT images should prompt careful review of the pleural reflection near the diaphragm, since finding talc deposits on the CT images will provide correct identification of pleurodesis.

REFERENCES

1. Kwek BH, Aquino SL, Fischman AJ. Fluorodeoxyglucose positron emission tomography and CT after talc pleurodesis. *Chest* 2004; **125**(6): 2356–2360.
2. Peek H, van der Bruggen W, Limonard G. Pleural FDG uptake more than a decade after talc pleurodesis. *Case Report Med* 2009; 2009: 650864.
3. Subramaniam RM, Wilcox B, Aubry MC, Jett J, Peller PJ. 18F-fluoro-2-deoxy D-glucose positron emission tomography and positron emission tomography/computed tomography imaging of malignant pleural mesothelioma. *J Med Imaging Radiat Oncol* 2009; **53**(2): 160–169.

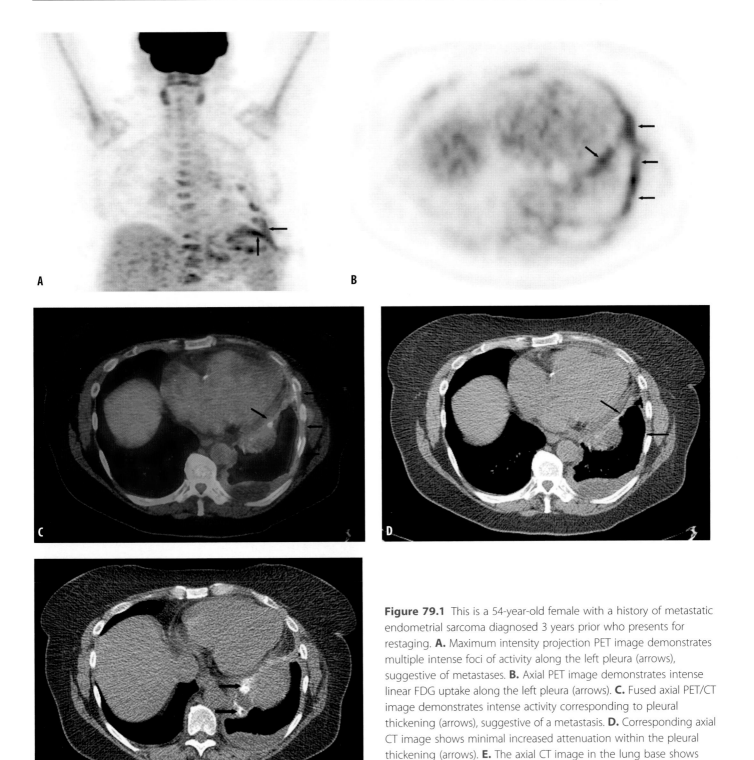

Figure 79.1 This is a 54-year-old female with a history of metastatic endometrial sarcoma diagnosed 3 years prior who presents for restaging. **A.** Maximum intensity projection PET image demonstrates multiple intense foci of activity along the left pleura (arrows), suggestive of metastases. **B.** Axial PET image demonstrates intense linear FDG uptake along the left pleura (arrows). **C.** Fused axial PET/CT image demonstrates intense activity corresponding to pleural thickening (arrows), suggestive of a metastasis. **D.** Corresponding axial CT image shows minimal increased attenuation within the pleural thickening (arrows). **E.** The axial CT image in the lung base shows dense talc deposits (arrows) and confirms talc pleurodesis as the cause of the left pleural abnormalities.

Esophagitis on PET/CT

Patrick Peller

Imaging description

In gastroesophageal reflux disease, the esophageal mucosa is subjected to chronic repetitive injury. The degree of inflammation is proportional to the frequency and duration of reflux events. Chronic reflux damage to the lower esophagus leads to replacement of the normal squamous cell lining with secretory columnar epithelium, which can withstand the erosive action of the gastric secretions. This metaplasia is termed Barrett's esophagus and confers an increased risk of adenocarcinoma. There is no relationship between the severity of reflux symptoms and the development of Barrett's esophagus. FDG uptake in distal esophageal inflammation, metaplasia, and early adenocarcinoma can be mild. Linear uptake is more common with benign causes of increased uptake (Figure 80.1) while focal and eccentric FDG uptake is associated with a higher rate of esophageal cancer at endoscopic biopsy (Figure 80.2) [1–3].

Importance

Reflux disease and Barrett's esophagus are common in the US and on PET/CT can resemble early esophageal malignancies. The challenge is to detect the incidental or synchronous esophageal carcinoma early while avoiding false positives from metaplasia and inflammation.

Typical clinical scenario

The patient is undergoing a PET/CT scan for evaluation of a condition unrelated to the esophagus. Increased FDG accumulation is noted incidentally in the distal esophagus. This activity can be due to inflammation, metaplasia, or neoplastic transformation. The dilemma is when should endoscopy be recommended.

Differential diagnosis

There is significant overlap of the FDG accumulation caused by benign esophagitis, dysplasia, and esophageal cancer. With intense FDG accumulation, eccentric and focal, rather than linear, uptake should prompt evaluation for malignant and premalignant disease. The combination of focal FDG uptake with eccentricity can differentiate those lesions that should undergo endoscopic evaluation to exclude malignancy.

> ### Teaching point
>
> Moderate to intense FDG accumulation in the distal esophagus can be secondary to esophagitis, Barrett's esophagus, and esophageal cancer. Focal, eccentric esophageal activity requires endoscopic evaluation.

REFERENCES

1. Israel O, Yefremov N, Bar-Shalom R, et al. PET/CT detection of unexpected gastrointestinal foci of 18F-FDG uptake: incidence, localization patterns, and clinical significance. *J Nucl Med* 2005; **46**(5): 758–762.
2. Kamel EM, Thumshirn M, Truninger K, et al. Significance of incidental 18F-FDG accumulations in the gastrointestinal tract in PET/CT: correlation with endoscopic and histopathologic results. *J Nucl Med* 2004; **45**(11): 1804–1810.
3. Roedl JB, Colen RR, King K, et al. Visual PET/CT scoring for nonspecific 18F-FDG uptake in the differentiation of early malignant and benign esophageal lesions. *AJR Am J Roentgenol* 2008; **191**(2): 515–521.

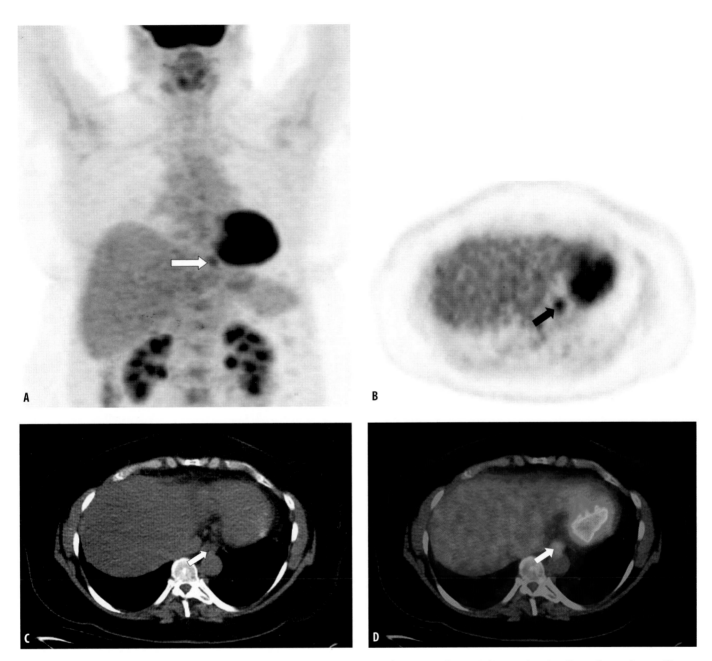

Figure 80.1 Man with a history of reflux disease diagnosed 3 years prior and recent endoscopic biopsy showing Barrett's esophagus. The PET/CT scan was performed to evaluate a new pulmonary nodule. **A.** Maximum intensity projection PET image demonstrates linear FDG activity in the distal esophagus (arrow) consistent with Barrett's esophagus. **B.** Axial PET image demonstrates moderate circumferential FDG uptake in the distal esophagus (arrow). **C.** Corresponding axial CT image shows mild, nonspecific thickening in the distal esophagus. **D.** Fused axial PET/CT image demonstrates the moderate activity corresponding to distal esophageal thickening (arrow), typical of esophagitis and Barrett's esophagus.

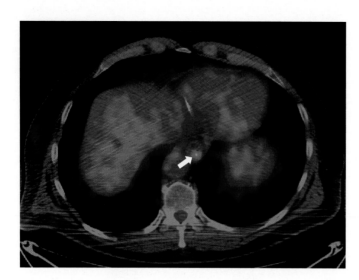

Figure 80.2 In a different patient, fused axial PET/CT image demonstrates focal, eccentric distal esophageal activity (arrow). Biopsy yielded a diagnosis of esophageal cancer.

Takayasu's arteritis on PET/CT

Patrick Peller

Imaging description

Takayasu's arteritis is a chronic vasculitis of unknown etiology, which primarily affects the aorta and its primary branches. Fever, malaise, and weight loss are the most common symptoms. Takayasu's arteritis primarily afflicts women and Asians. The arteritis may be localized to a segment of any large artery or may involve the aorta and multiple vessels contiguously [1–3]. PET/CT demonstrates intense FDG uptake within the thickened, inflamed arterial walls (Figure 81.1). PET/CT is more sensitive than CT and MRI in detecting disease extent and identifying segmental arteritis. PET/CT can distinguish vessel thickening due to fibrosis from active inflammation. FDG uptake correlates with clinical markers of inflammation and can be used to evaluate response to therapy [4].

Importance

Takayasu's arteritis often presents with nonspecific clinical findings, often suggestive of an underlying malignancy. Overlooking the diffuse arterial wall activity can lead to adverse consequences for the patient. The moderate to intense linear FDG accumulation within the walls of the great vessels should not be confused as secondary to atherosclerotic disease.

Typical clinical scenario

Constitutional symptoms with or without ischemic symptoms in a woman younger than 40 years should raise a suspicion for

Takayasu's arteritis. Blood work showing a highly elevated erythrocyte sedimentation rate should trigger urgent imaging.

Differential diagnosis

The imaging features of Takayasu's arteritis on PET/CT are relatively characteristic with linear FDG uptake in the thickened arterial walls. The involvement of carotid, subclavian, aortic, and iliac walls with homogeneous FDG accumulation is common. Atherosclerotic disease in the elderly, especially males, can have mild uptake irregularly, usually within aortic and iliac walls. The mild diffuse FDG uptake is also seen in vascular grafts.

> ## Teaching point
>
> Linear and intense FDG accumulation within the walls of the large arteries is typical of Takayasu's arteritis on PET/CT.

REFERENCES

1. Lupi-Herrera E, Sanchez-Torres G, Marcushamer J, et al. Takayasu's arteritis. Clinical study of 107 cases. *Am Heart J* 1977; **93**: 94–103.
2. Hall S, Barr W, Lie JT, et al. Takayasu arteritis: a study of 32 North American patients. *Medicine* 1985; **64**: 89–99.
3. Cid MC, Font C, Coll-VinentB, Grau JM. Large vessel vasculitides. *Curr Opin Rheumatol* 1998; **10**: 18–28.
4. Walter MA. [(18)F] fluorodeoxyglucose PET in large vessel vasculitis. *Radiol Clin North Am* 2007; **45**(4): 735–744.

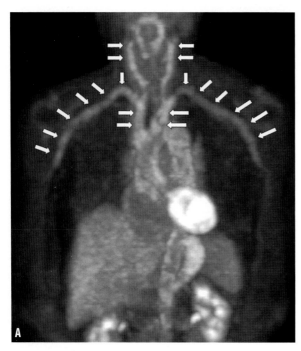

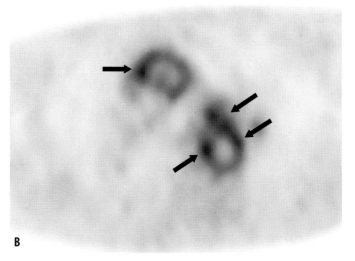

Figure 81.1 (cont.)

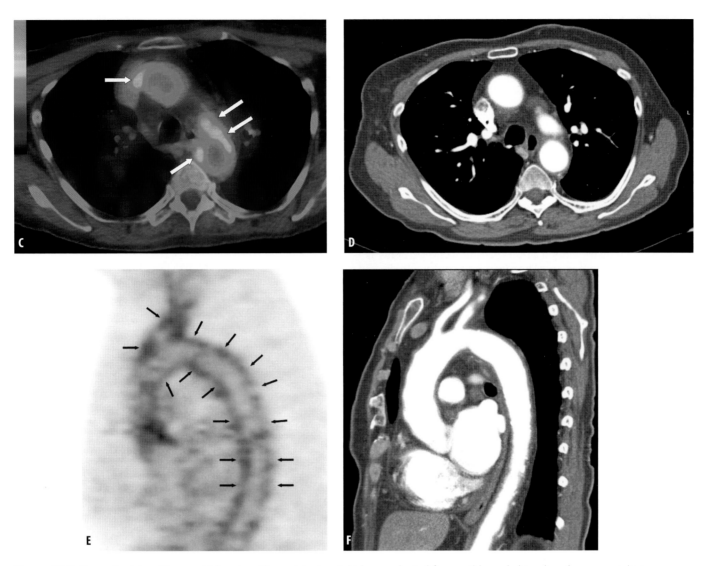

Figure 81.1 The patient is a 40-year-old female with persistent weight loss evaluated for possible underlying lymphoma or malignancy. **A.** Maximum intensity projection PET image demonstrates intense activity in the aortic walls extending into the carotid, subclavian, and axillary arteries symmetrically (arrows). **B.** Axial PET image demonstrates intense activity within the aortic arch (arrows). **C.** Fused axial PET/CT image demonstrates the intense activity lies within the aortic wall (arrows). **D.** Corresponding contrast-enhanced axial CT image shows near-symmetrical wall thickening in the aortic arch. **E.** Sagittal PET image shows linear, intense activity in the ascending aorta continuing into the carotid artery and throughout the entire descending thoracic aorta (arrows), typical of Takayasu's arteritis. **F.** Corresponding contrast-enhanced sagittal CT image shows thickened arterial walls throughout the entire descending thoracic aorta.

Window and level settings

Thomas Hartman

Imaging description

Window and level settings can significantly affect the appearance of CT images. Therefore, over time, relatively standard window and level settings have been established for evaluation of the lungs, soft tissues, and bones. However, there are occasions when alteration of the window and level settings may be helpful in diagnosis of disease.

Alteration of window and level settings may be helpful in detecting pulmonary emboli [1]. When the contrast bolus is very dense, small emboli may be obscured on a standard soft tissue (mediastinal) window and level setting (Figure 82.1). By narrowing the window and level settings, the embolus can be more easily detected (Figure 82.1). Narrow CT window widths can also be useful in detecting subtle emphysema [2, 3]. However, care must be taken in evaluating other structures in the chest since narrow CT window widths – especially when combined with low level settings – can simulate the appearance of infiltrative lung disease or bronchial wall thickening [2, 3].

Importance

Studies are routinely evaluated at typical window and level settings and this is helpful to minimize artificially altering the appearance of bronchial walls or the lung parenchyma. However, there are times that alteration of the window and level settings may be beneficial. This should only be done for specific indications and the remainder of the exam should be viewed with the standard window and level settings.

Typical clinical scenario

When the indication for the CT exam is emphysema or pulmonary embolism, it may be appropriate to alter the window and level settings in these instances.

Differential diagnosis

There is no differential diagnosis, but be aware that alteration of the window and level settings can result in misrepresentation of bronchial wall thickening or interstitial lung disease. Therefore, alteration of the window and level settings should only be done for a few specific indications.

Teaching point

It is important to evaluate the lungs using consistent window and level settings to prevent artificially altering the appearance of the lung parenchyma or bronchial walls. However, for the detection of pulmonary emboli or subtle emphysema alteration of the typical window and level settings may be beneficial.

REFERENCES
1. Brink JA, Woodard PK, Horesh L, et al. Depiction of pulmonary emboli with spiral CT: optimization of display window settings in a porcine model. *Radiology* 1997; **204**: 703–708.
2. Bankier AA, Fleischmann D, Mallek R, et al. Bronchial wall thickness: appropriate window settings for thin-section CT and radiologic-anatomic correlation. *Radiology* 1996; **199**: 831–836.
3. Primack SL, Remy-Jardin M, Remy J, Müller NL. High-resolution CT of the lung: pitfalls in the diagnosis of infiltrative lung disease. *AJR Am J Roentgenol* 1996; **167**: 413–418.

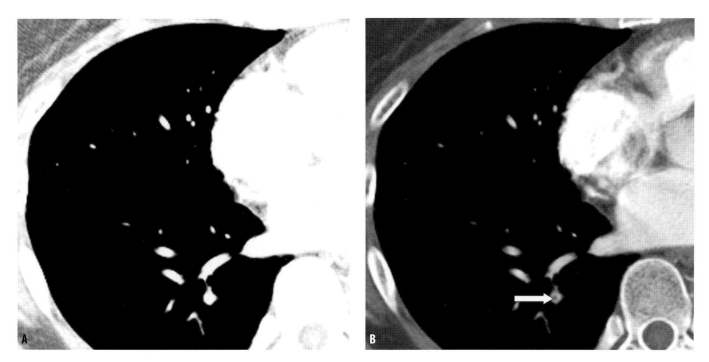

Figure 82.1 **A.** CT chest with intravenous contrast performed for evaluation of pulmonary emboli. Targeted view of the right lung with "standard" window and level settings. No pulmonary emboli are detected. **B.** CT chest with intravenous contrast performed for evaluation of pulmonary emboli. Targeted view of the right lung with narrower window and level settings than in Figure 82.1A. A pulmonary embolus is seen in a subsegmental branch of the right lower lobe pulmonary artery (arrow).

Stair step artifacts

Anne-Marie Sykes

Imaging description

Stair step artifact is seen on multiplanar (coronal and sagittal) and three-dimensional reformatted CT images, when wide collimations and nonoverlapping reconstruction intervals are used [1]. It is seen as low-attenuation lines around the edges or traversing vessels, giving them the appearance of a series of steps. This artifact is more pronounced when wide collimations and nonoverlapping reconstruction intervals are used. The artifact is accentuated by cardiac and respiratory motion (Figure 83.1).

Importance

Failure to recognize this artifact could result in a misdiagnosis of pulmonary embolism.

Typical clinical scenario

This artifact results when sagittal and coronal reformatted images are produced without overlap of the raw data. It is accentuated by cardiac and respiratory motion.

Differential diagnosis

The main differential diagnosis is pulmonary embolism. Additional considerations include other artifacts such as beam-hardening or streak artifact.

Teaching point

Stair step artifact can be reduced or eliminated by reconstructing the raw data with a 50% overlap prior to image reconstruction [2]. This artifact will not be completely eliminated when it is due to cardiac or respiratory motion artifact. Scanning on the faster generation CT scans results in a decrease in these motion artifacts.

REFERENCES

1. Barret JF, Keat N. Artifacts in CT: recognition and avoidance. *Radiographics* 2004; **24**: 1679–1691.
2. Wittram C, Maher MM, Yoo AJ, et al. CT angiography of pulmonary embolism: diagnostic criteria and causes of misdiagnosis. *Radiographics* 2004; **24**: 1219–1238.

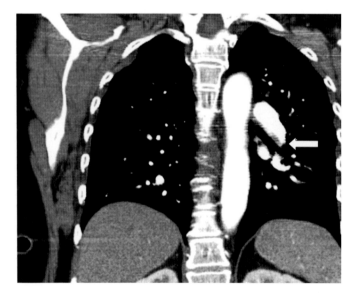

Figure 83.1 Stair step artifact. Coronal reformatted images from a PE study, with irregularity of the margins of the vessels (arrow), giving the appearance of steps on a stairway.

Streak artifacts

Anne-Marie Sykes

Imaging description

In very heterogeneous cross sections, dark (low-attenuation) bands or streaks can appear between two dense objects in an image. They occur because the portion of the beam that passes through one of the objects at certain tube positions is hardened less than when it passes through both objects at other tube positions [1]. This type of artifact can occur in bony regions of the body; in scans where contrast medium has been used; and from lines, devices, and surgical clips. The artifact is usually nonanatomic, poorly defined, and radiating [2].

Importance

Streak artifacts from dense contrast in the superior vena cava (SVC) are common, and can be seen overlying the right main and right upper lobe pulmonary arteries. These areas of decreased attenuation can be mistaken for intraluminal filling defects (Figure 84.1), or they could obscure the vessels for accurate assessment for pulmonary embolism. Similar artifacts arise from pacemaker leads, surgical clips, or similar structures.

Typical clinical scenario

A diagnostic CT pulmonary embolism study requires good opacification of the pulmonary arteries, and the bolus of

intravenous contrast in the SVC is usually quite dense. This can result in a beam-hardening streak artifact, with low-attenuation streaks radiating out from the SVC.

Differential diagnosis

The main differential diagnosis is pulmonary embolism. Other considerations include other artifacts such as stair step artifact.

> ### Teaching point
>
> Streak artifact should be recognized by its nonanatomic, poorly defined, and radiating nature. Streak artifact from dense contrast in the SVC can be diminished by saline flush of the SVC using dual-chamber injectors.

REFERENCES

1. Barret JF, Keat N. Artifacts in CT: recognition and avoidance. *Radiographics* 2004; **24**: 1679–1691.
2. Wittram C, Maher MM, Yoo AJ, et al. CT angiography of pulmonary embolism: diagnostic criteria and causes of misdiagnosis. *Radiographics* 2004; **24**: 1219–1238.

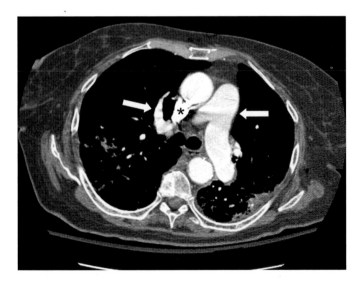

Figure 84.1 Streak artifact. A band of low attenuation is seen over the bifurcation of the central pulmonary arteries (arrows) due to beam-hardening artifact from the very dense contrast in the SVC (asterisk). Note the non-anatomic, poorly defined radiating nature of the streaks.

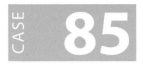

Respiratory motion

Anne-Marie Sykes

Imaging description

Acute and chronic pulmonary emboli (PE) on contrast-enhanced CT chest are recognized as intraluminal filling defects within opacified pulmonary arteries. The filling defects may be complete or partial. The interface with intravenous contrast material should be sharp. Respiratory motion artifact may result in apparent termination of vessels or result in volume averaging with surrounding air-filled lung, mimicking an intraluminal filling defect [1]. and could be misinterpreted as a pulmonary embolus (Figure 85.1).

Importance

Annually, as many as 300000 people in the United States die from acute pulmonary embolism [2]. Most of the deaths from PE result from failure of diagnosis rather than from treatment failure [3]. However, overdiagnosis of PE should also be avoided as there can be complications associated with the treatment of PE. Anticoagulation is the main therapy for acute PE. It is estimated that major bleeding (intracranial hemorrhage, retroperitoneal hemorrhage, or bleeding that led directly to death, hospitalization, or transfusion) occurs in fewer than 3% of patients receiving intravenous unfractionated heparin or oral warfarin to treat PE or deep vein thrombosis [4]. Heparin-induced thrombocytopenia (HIT) is another complication of heparin therapy.

In addition to striving to diagnose pulmonary embolism on CT, the radiologist should try to avoid pitfalls in falsely diagnosing PE when none are present.

Typical clinical scenario

A good PE CT study is one that optimally opacifies and demonstrates the main, lobar, segmental, and subsegmental arteries in all lobes. The patient in whom pulmonary embolism is suspected is generally short of breath, and may not be able to hold his/her breath for the duration of the scan. The resulting motion can cause an averaging of the densities of the involved structures. In this case, the density of the opacified pulmonary vessel (high attenuation) is averaged with the density of the lung (very low attenuation), and the result is an apparent area of low attenuation within the vessel at the affected level.

Differential diagnosis

The main differential diagnosis is bland pulmonary thromboembolic disease.

> ### Teaching point
>
> Unlike true PE, the low density "filling defect" from respiratory motion artifact does *not* make a sharp interface with the intravenous contrast. The radiologist should always look at the lung window settings. Respiratory motion is shown as blurring of the vessels, with composite images of the vessels (the seagull sign). This motion artifact renders the diagnosis of PE at this anatomic level indeterminate.

REFERENCES

1. Rémy-Jardin M, Rémy J, Mayo JR, Müller NL. *CT Angiography of the Chest.* Philadelphia, PA: Lippincott Williams & Wilkins, 2001.
2. Tapson VF. Acute pulmonary embolism. *N Engl J Med* 2008; **358**: 1037–1052.
3. Zhang, L-J, Zhao Y-E, Wu S-Y, et al. Pulmonary embolism detection with dual-energy CT: experimental study of dual source CT in rabbits. *Radiology* 2009; **252**: 61–70.
4. Schulman S, Beyth RJ, Kearon C, Levine MN. Hemorrhagic complications of anticoagulant and thrombolytic treatment: American College of Chest Physicians Evidence-Based Clinical Practice Guidelines (8th Edition). *Chest* 2008; **133**(6 Suppl): 257S–298S.

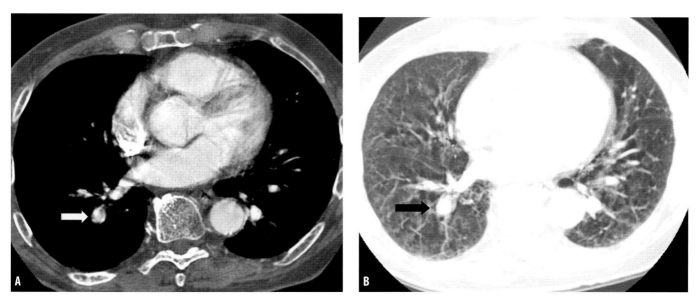

Figure 85.1 **A.** Low density within the right lower lobe pulmonary artery (arrow) mimics a filling defect (pseudo-filling defect). Note that the interface with the intravenous contrast material is not sharp. **B.** Lung windows at the same level show extensive respiratory motion artifact, with blurring of vessels as well as the "seagull sign" (composite images of the vessels).

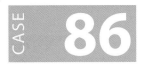
86 Lung reconstruction algorithm

Anne-Marie Sykes

Imaging description

The lung algorithm is a high-spatial-frequency reconstruction convolution kernel that results in edge enhancement and is used to improve the quality of the lung images and show fine anatomic structures on CT [1]. However, an additional result of edge enhancement is that on CT the margin of the pulmonary artery will be of higher attenuation than the central portion (bright ring around the vessel) (Figure 86.1).

Importance

The higher attenuation margin of a pulmonary artery can mimic the appearance of pulmonary emboli, particularly if it is associated with flow artifact (poor contrast opacification of the vessel).

Typical clinical scenario

If the radiologist inadvertently views the mediastinal or pulmonary embolism-specific (vascular) windows with a lung algorithm, edge enhancement of the vessels will occur, and could result in misinterpretation as positive for pulmonary embolism.

Differential diagnosis

The main differential diagnosis is pulmonary embolism.

Teaching point

Ensure that the appropriate algorithm is obtained. This artifact can be removed using a standard algorithm [2].

REFERENCES
1. Wittram C, Maher MM, Yoo AJ, et al. CT angiography of pulmonary embolism: diagnostic criteria and causes of misdiagnosis. *Radiographics* 2004; **24**: 1219–1238.
2. Gosselin MV, Rassner UA, Thieszen SL, et al. Contrast dynamics during CT pulmonary angiogram: analysis of an inspiration associated artifact. *J Thorac Imaging* 2004; **19**: 1–7.

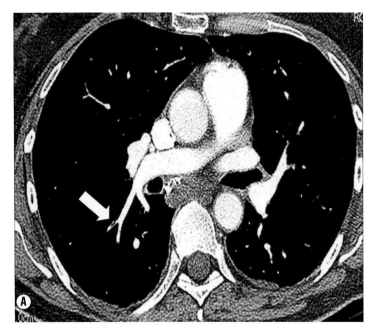
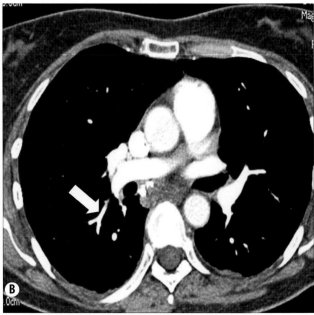

Figure 86.1 **A.** High-spatial-frequency algorithm – apparent intraluminal filling defect in a branch of the right lower lobe pulmonary artery (white arrow), due to edge enhancement. **B.** Same image using standard algorithm shows no filling defect in the artery (white arrow).

Index